The Complete Anti-inflammatory Diet for Women

A Comprehensive Formula to Reducing Inflammation, Boosting Health, and Thriving in Every Stage of Life.

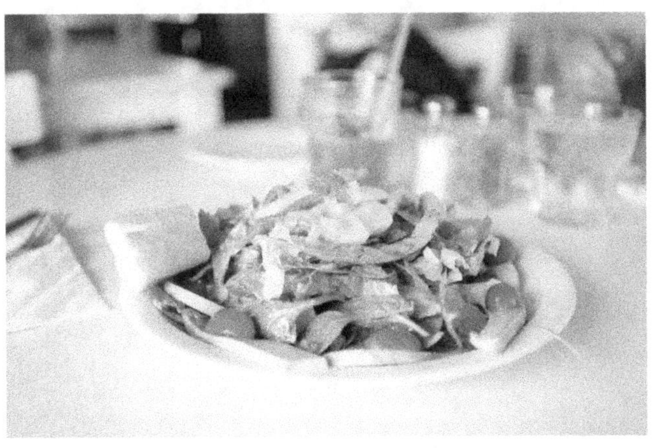

By
Dovie Betty

TABLE OF CONTENTS

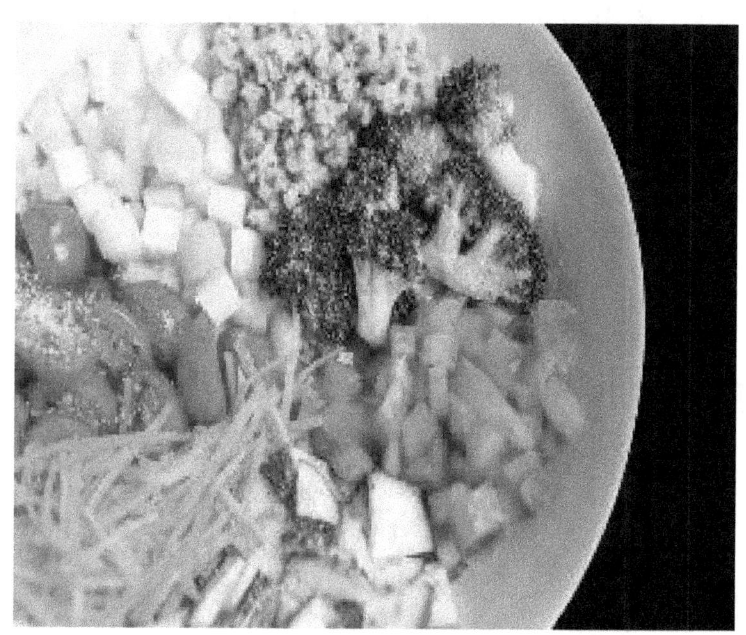

Introduction

In the heart of a bustling city, where life's pace often feels like a never-ending sprint, I found myself juggling a demanding career, a family to care for, and the incessant demands of daily life. Like many women, I felt pulled in every direction, my well-being often pushed to the back burner. It was a familiar story of modern womanhood, and I was no exception.

Amidst this whirlwind, I encountered a health challenge that would forever change the trajectory of my life. It was a diagnosis of chronic inflammation, something that, like countless others, I had never truly understood until it affected me personally. This inflammation manifested itself in mysterious aches, persistent fatigue, and an overall sense of unease. It was as if my body was sending distress signals, and I had no choice but to listen.

In my quest for answers and healing, I dove headfirst into the world of anti-inflammatory living. It was a journey of discovery, filled with ups and downs, experimentation, and, ultimately, transformation. Through dietary changes, lifestyle adjustments, and a newfound understanding of how inflammation impacts women uniquely, I began to reclaim my health and vitality. It was a journey that empowered me, not just as a woman but as an advocate for my own well-being.

As I delved deeper into the science behind inflammation and nutrition, I realized that I wasn't alone in this struggle. Many women were facing similar challenges, battling the silent inflammation that lurked within their bodies. The more I learned, the more I felt compelled to share this knowledge, to guide and support other women on their path to vibrant health.

And so, this book was born a comprehensive guide to "The Complete Anti-Inflammatory Diet for Women." It's not just a compilation of scientific facts and dietary advice; it's a reflection of my own journey and the countless women I've had the privilege to help along the way.

Within these pages, you'll find a roadmap to understanding inflammation, embracing a diet rich in healing foods, and adopting a lifestyle that promotes wellness at every stage of life. Whether you're a young woman looking to proactively safeguard your health, a mother seeking vitality to care for your family, or a woman entering a new chapter of life, this book is designed to empower you.

Together, I'll explore the science behind inflammation, discover the power of food as medicine, and embark on a journey to greater health and wellness. I invite you to join me on this transformative adventure—a journey that has the potential to change not only your health but also your life.

So, let's begin. It's time to nourish your body, relieve inflammation, and thrive in health and wellness.

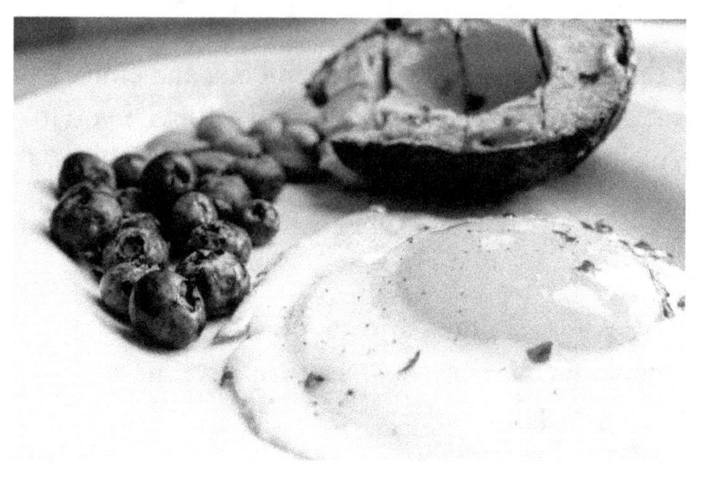

Chapter 1: Understanding Inflammation

In the intricate symphony of the human body, inflammation is both a lifesaver and a potential disruptor of harmony. Like a double-edged sword, inflammation plays a vital role in our body's defense mechanisms, yet when it becomes chronic, it can wreak havoc on our health. To embark on our journey towards a complete anti-inflammatory diet for women, it's imperative that we first grasp the fundamental concept of inflammation.

In this chapter, I'll dive deep into the world of inflammation, unraveling its mysteries and gaining a clear understanding of its impact on our bodies. I'll explore the difference between acute and chronic inflammation, learn about the intricate web of signals that trigger an inflammatory response, and uncover the reasons why inflammation matters significantly in the context of women's health.

As I navigate this exploration, I'll lay the foundation for the rest of our journey. By the end of this chapter, you'll have a solid grasp of the science behind inflammation and its potential implications for your well-being. Armed with this knowledge, you'll be better equipped to make informed choices about your diet and lifestyle, setting the stage for your transformative path toward a healthier and more vibrant you. So, let's begin our exploration of understanding inflammation, the cornerstone of your journey towards a complete anti-inflammatory diet for women.

What Is Inflammation?

In the complex and finely tuned orchestra of the human body, inflammation is a powerful, natural response that plays a crucial role in protecting us from harm and aiding in healing. It is a biological reaction that occurs when our body senses an injury, infection, or other forms of damage. While this acute inflammatory response is essential for our survival, it's important to distinguish it from the chronic inflammation that can silently undermine our health.

The Dance of Acute Inflammation

Imagine this scenario: you accidentally cut your finger while slicing vegetables in the kitchen. Almost instantly, your body leaps into action to protect and heal the wounded area. This is acute inflammation in action.

Key characteristics of acute inflammation include:

Redness: Blood vessels near the injury dilate, causing the area to become red and warm. This increased blood flow carries immune cells and nutrients to the site of injury.

Swelling: Fluid and white blood cells rush to the injured area, causing swelling. This swelling helps immobilize the affected area and protect it from further damage.

Heat: Increased blood flow not only brings immune cells but also warmth. The warmth is a sign of inflammation at work.

Pain: Pain receptors in the area become more sensitive, alerting you to the injury. This pain discourages you from further damaging the injured area.

Loss of Function: In some cases, inflammation can temporarily limit the function of the injured area to prevent additional harm.

This immediate and localized response is a fundamental part of our body's defense mechanism. Once the threat is neutralized, inflammation subsides, and the healing process continues. In acute situations like these, inflammation is a lifesaver.

The Perils of Chronic Inflammation

However, there is another side to inflammation—one that lingers, often unnoticed until it contributes to a cascade of health problems. This is chronic inflammation. Instead of a short-lived and focused response, chronic inflammation is a persistent, low-grade immune response that can affect the entire body. Unlike acute inflammation, which serves a protective purpose, chronic inflammation can harm healthy tissues and cells.

Several factors, including the following, can contribute to chronic inflammation:

Diet: Consuming foods high in sugar, trans fats, and processed ingredients can trigger inflammation.

Lifestyle: Smoking, excessive alcohol consumption, lack of exercise, and chronic stress can all contribute to chronic inflammation.

Environmental Toxins: Exposure to pollutants, chemicals, and allergens can promote inflammation.

Disease: Certain diseases and conditions, such as obesity, autoimmune disorders, and chronic infections, can perpetuate inflammation.

Why is this distinction between acute and chronic inflammation important for women's health? Because chronic inflammation has been linked to a range of health issues that disproportionately affect women, including autoimmune diseases, heart disease, cancer, and reproductive health challenges.

Understanding the delicate balance between these two types of inflammation is crucial on our journey toward a complete anti-inflammatory diet for women. It empowers us to make informed dietary and lifestyle choices that can help reduce chronic inflammation and promote our well-being. In the chapters that follow, w
I'll explore how foods, lifestyle adjustments, and mindful choices can aid us in the pursuit of vibrant health and vitality. But first, let's delve even deeper into the science behind inflammation and its intricate relationship with our immune system and overall health.

The Role of Chronic Inflammation in Women's Health

Chronic inflammation, once considered a silent intruder in the realm of health, has garnered significant attention in recent years. Its role in the development and progression of various diseases and its distinct impact on women's health cannot be underestimated. In this part, I'll delve into the intricate relationship between chronic inflammation and the well-being of women, shedding light on why it is a crucial consideration on our journey toward a complete anti-inflammatory diet for women.

The Gender Connection: Why Inflammation Matters More for Women

While inflammation affects both men and women, research suggests that women may be more susceptible to chronic inflammatory conditions. This gender disparity is not entirely understood, but it highlights the unique health challenges women face throughout their lives.

Autoimmune Diseases

Autoimmune diseases, a group of conditions where the immune system mistakenly attacks the body's own tissues, are more prevalent in women. Conditions like rheumatoid arthritis, lupus, multiple sclerosis, and Hashimoto's thyroiditis are examples of autoimmune diseases that disproportionately affect women. The exact reasons behind this gender disparity remain a subject of ongoing research, but hormones, genetic factors, and the interplay between the two are believed to play a role.

Hormonal Changes

Women experience distinct hormonal fluctuations throughout their lives, from menstruation and pregnancy to menopause. These hormonal shifts can influence the body's inflammatory responses. For example, the menstrual cycle can lead to cyclical changes in inflammation markers, potentially contributing to symptoms like menstrual cramps and mood swings. Additionally, the menopausal transition can bring about changes in inflammatory patterns that may impact a woman's health.

Fertility and Reproductive Health

Inflammation can also affect fertility and reproductive health. Conditions like polycystic ovary syndrome (PCOS) and endometriosis, which involve inflammation, are common culprits of fertility challenges in women. Understanding how inflammation influences these conditions is crucial for women seeking to conceive.

Inflammatory Impact on Women's Health Conditions

Beyond the gender-specific factors, chronic inflammation has been implicated in several health conditions that disproportionately affect women. These conditions include:

Heart Disease: Chronic inflammation can contribute to the development of atherosclerosis, a condition characterized by the buildup of plaque in arteries. Women with chronic inflammation may be at a higher risk of heart disease.

Cancer: Inflammation is associated with an increased risk of various types of cancer. This includes breast cancer, ovarian cancer, and cervical cancer. Reducing chronic inflammation may play a preventive role in these cancers.

Mood Disorders: Inflammation can impact mood and mental health. Conditions like depression and anxiety have been linked to chronic inflammation, and women are more likely to experience these mood disorders.

Autoimmune Diseases: As mentioned earlier, many autoimmune diseases are more prevalent in women. These conditions can be painful and debilitating, significantly impacting a woman's quality of life.

Understanding the profound effect of chronic inflammation on women's health underscores the importance of addressing it proactively. In the upcoming chapters, I will explore the dietary and lifestyle changes that can help manage and reduce inflammation, empowering women to take charge of their health and well-being. By harnessing the power of an anti-inflammatory diet, we can pave the way to a healthier, more vibrant future, where inflammation no longer holds us back from living life to the fullest.

Identifying Inflammatory Triggers

Now that I've established the critical role of inflammation in women's health, the next step on our journey to a complete anti-inflammatory diet for women is to identify the triggers that can set off this chronic inflammatory response. Understanding these triggers empowers us to make informed choices about our lifestyle, diet, and overall well-being.

Dietary Inflammatory Triggers

Our diet has a profound impact on inflammation. Some dietary choices can fuel chronic inflammation, while others can help combat it. Here are common dietary inflammatory triggers to be aware of:

Sugars and Refined Carbohydrates: Foods high in sugars and refined carbohydrates, such as white bread, sugary snacks, and sweetened beverages, can lead to spikes in blood sugar levels and promote inflammation.

Trans Fats: Artificial trans fats, often found in partially hydrogenated oils used in processed and fried foods, have been strongly linked to inflammation and various health problems.

Saturated Fats: While not inherently inflammatory, excessive consumption of saturated fats, especially from sources like red meat and full-fat dairy, can contribute to inflammation when not balanced with anti-inflammatory foods.

Omega-6 Fatty Acids: These fatty acids, found in vegetable oils like corn, soybean, and sunflower oil, can promote inflammation when consumed in excess, especially when not balanced with omega-3 fatty acids.

Food Sensitivities: Individual food sensitivities can trigger an inflammatory response in the body. Common culprits include gluten, dairy, and certain nightshade vegetables.

Lifestyle and Environmental Triggers

Beyond diet, various lifestyle and environmental factors can also contribute to chronic inflammation

Stress: Chronic stress can lead to the release of stress hormones and inflammatory molecules in the body, promoting inflammation over time.

Lack of Physical Activity: Sedentary lifestyles can contribute to chronic inflammation. Regular physical activity has anti-inflammatory effects.

Smoking: Smoking is a known pro-inflammatory factor that can harm various organs and systems in the body.

Excessive Alcohol Consumption: Heavy drinking can trigger inflammation and negatively impact the liver.

Environmental Toxins: Exposure to pollutants, chemicals, and allergens in the environment can promote inflammation in sensitive individuals.

Identifying Your Personal Triggers

It's important to recognize that inflammatory triggers can vary from person to person. What may cause inflammation in one individual might not affect another in the same way. This highlights the importance of personalized approaches to dietary and lifestyle choices.

Keeping a Food Diary: If you suspect certain foods may be triggering inflammation for you, consider keeping a food diary. Record what you eat and how you feel afterward to identify patterns.

Consulting a Healthcare Professional: If you have persistent health issues or suspect food sensitivities, consider consulting a healthcare professional, such as a registered dietitian or allergist, for testing and guidance.

Lifestyle Assessment: Reflect on your lifestyle choices, stress levels, and environmental exposures to identify potential triggers for chronic inflammation.

Identifying and addressing your specific inflammatory triggers is a significant step toward adopting an anti-inflammatory diet and lifestyle. Armed with this knowledge, you can make targeted changes that will have a positive impact on your health and well-being. In the chapters ahead, I will explore how to replace inflammatory triggers with anti-inflammatory solutions, setting you on the path to a healthier, more vibrant life.

Chapter 2: The Science Behind the Anti-Inflammatory Diet

It is essential to establish a solid understanding foundation in our endeavor to adopt a comprehensive anti-inflammatory diet designed specifically for women's health. The anti-inflammatory diet's principles, mechanisms, and evidence are examined in this chapter, which takes us on a journey into the fascinating field of nutritional science.

But why is it so important to look into the science behind this diet? Information is the compass that directs our excursion, empowering us to pursue informed decisions and really value the groundbreaking force of the mitigating diet. I will learn the reasons why certain foods can either stoke inflammation or put an end to it in our bodies as we begin this investigation.

So, let's take a look at the science behind the anti-inflammatory diet and learn how to use food as a medicine for women's health to its fullest potential. To unlock the keys to a life that is both healthier and more vibrant, it is time to dissect the connection between the foods we eat and inflammation.

Inflammation and Disease: Connecting the Dots

Inflammation is a biological response that is meant to heal and protect the intricate fabric of the human body. However, it can set the stage for a wide range of diseases when this finely tuned mechanism becomes chronically dysfunctional. As I investigate the science behind the anti-inflammatory diet, it is essential to comprehend the intricate connection between inflammation and these health conditions.

The Inflammatory Cascade It is essential to comprehend the sequence of events that take place within the body when inflammation is triggered in order to comprehend the connection between inflammation and disease.
Here is an improved on outline:

Trigger: When the body senses an injury, infection, or irritant, inflammation typically begins. To alert the immune system, cells release chemical signals known as cytokines.

Immune Reaction: In order to eliminate the threat, the immune system sends immune cells to the site of inflammation. This prompts the trademark indications of irritation — redness, enlarging, warmth, and agony.

Process of Healing: When the danger is contained or wiped out, the body's mending cycle starts. In cases of acute inflammation, this typically results in complete healing.

However, this cycle can become self-perpetuating in chronic inflammation, requiring the immune system to remain alert at all times. Various diseases and collateral damage to healthy tissues can result from this persistent inflammation.

Disease and Chronic Inflammation Chronic inflammation has been linked to a wide range of diseases, many of which are more prevalent in women. Let's look at a few important health conditions in which inflammation plays a crucial role:

Diseases of the Heart: Ongoing irritation can harm veins and advance the arrangement of blood vessel plaque. This has the potential to raise the risk of heart disease, including strokes and heart attacks, over time.

Conditions of Autoimmunity: The immune system mistakenly attacks the body's own tissues in conditions like rheumatoid arthritis, lupus, and multiple sclerosis. Autoimmune conditions are characterized by persistent inflammation.

Leukemia: An environment that is favorable to the growth and spread of cancer cells can be created by inflammation. Breast and colon cancer, among others, have been linked to chronic inflammation.

Diabetes and metabolic syndrome: Insulin resistance, the development of metabolic syndrome, and type 2 diabetes are all linked to chronic inflammation.

Neurodegenerative Illnesses: Inflammation is a component of diseases like Alzheimer's and Parkinson's that may accelerate disease progression.

Conditions of the womb: Endometriosis and polycystic ovary syndrome (PCOS), which are prevalent in women, can be made worse by chronic inflammation.

We learn more about the significant impact that chronic inflammation has on women's health by connecting the dots between these health conditions and inflammation. It emphasizes the urgency of adopting a diet and lifestyle that are anti-inflammatory to lower the risk of these diseases and improve overall health.

Women who want to improve their health and vitality will find hope and empowerment in the chapters that follow as I examine the aspects of diet and lifestyle that can reduce chronic inflammation.

The Immune System and Inflammation

The immune system orchestrates responses that shield us from pathogens, injuries, and foreign invaders in the complex symphony of the human body. As I investigate the science behind the anti-inflammatory diet for women, it is essential to comprehend how the immune system reacts to inflammation.

The Body's Defenses: The immune system is a complex network of cells, tissues, and organs that work together to protect our health. Its main job is to find and kill anything foreign that gets into our bodies, like bacteria, viruses, fungi, or other dangers. This insusceptible reaction is fundamental for our endurance.

The Resistant Framework's Part in Aggravation

Aggravation and the safe framework are unpredictably connected. In point of fact, a common immune system response to a perceived threat is inflammation. This connection works as follows:

Recognition: An inflammatory response is triggered when the immune system detects a potential threat. Immune cells known as macrophages, which serve as sentinels and search tissues for indications of trouble, may initiate this.

Compound Signs: These alerted sentinel cells release cytokines, chemical signals. Similar to messengers, these cytokines instruct other immune cells to join the fight.

Recruitment of Immune Cells: These signals cause immune cells, such as white blood cells and neutrophils, to migrate to the site of inflammation. The most recognizable symptoms of inflammation result from this recruitment: pain, redness, swelling, and warmth

Neutralization: The elimination of the threat—whether it be a bacterium, a virus, or damaged tissue—is the ultimate objective of the immune system. The immune system stops responding to a threat in acute inflammation.

However, this response can become persistent in chronic inflammation, keeping the immune system on constant alert. As previously mentioned, this ongoing immune activation can result in a series of health issues.

Women's Health and the Immune System The immune system's role in women's health goes beyond infection prevention. Reproductive health, pregnancy, and hormonal regulation all depend on it. Sex hormones like estrogen and progesterone have an impact on the unique patterns and responses that women's immune systems exhibit. During the menstrual cycle and during pregnancy, these hormonal fluctuations may influence inflammatory responses.

Women who want to improve their health and well-being by following an anti-inflammatory diet need to have a solid understanding of the intricate connection that exists between the immune system, inflammation, and hormonal fluctuations.

As I dive further into the science behind the mitigating diet in the accompanying sections, I will investigate how dietary decisions can regulate the safe framework's reactions and add to the administration of ongoing irritation. Women can make informed dietary choices that support immune health as well as overall vitality and wellness with this knowledge.

Foods that Fuel Inflammation vs. Foods that Fight It

The choices we make at the dinner table can have significant effects on our health because of the intricate relationship between diet and inflammation. Inflammation is known to be fueled by some foods, while others have anti-inflammatory properties that can help reduce chronic inflammation. Women will gain the knowledge they need to make educated choices regarding their nutrition as a result of this section's in-depth examination of the scientific basis for these dietary choices.

Root Causes of Inflammation: Foods that Inflame and Cause Inflammation

Refined and Sugary Carbohydrates: High-sugar counts calories and refined starches, like those tracked down in sweet tidbits, cakes, and improved drinks, can prompt fast spikes in glucose levels. This flood sets off the arrival of incendiary cytokines.

Trans fats: The infamous inflammatory effects of artificial trans fats, which can be found in processed and fried foods, are well-known. They advance aggravation as well as increment the gamble of coronary illness and other medical problems.

Saturated Fats: While not intrinsically provocative, over the top utilization of soaked fats, frequently obtained from red meat and full-fat dairy, can add to aggravation when not offset with calming food varieties.

Omega-6 Unsaturated fats: Omega-6 fatty acids are necessary for health and are mostly found in vegetable oils like corn, soybean, and sunflower oil. However, inflammation may be exacerbated by an excess of omega-6 fatty acids and an imbalance between omega-3 and omega-6 fatty acids.

Red and processed meats: Red meats like beef and pork, as well as processed meats like sausages, contain compounds that, when consumed in large quantities, can cause inflammation.

Calming Legends: Foods that Reduce Inflammation Vegetables and Fruits: Antioxidants and phytochemicals that reduce inflammation are abundant in these nutritional powerhouses. Berries, broccoli, sweet potatoes, and leafy greens are excellent options.

Lean Meat: Omega-3 fatty acids are abundant in salmon, mackerel, sardines, and trout and have potent anti-inflammatory properties.

Seeds and Nuts: Healthy fats, fiber, and anti-inflammatory antioxidants are abundant in flaxseeds, chia seeds, almonds, and walnuts.

Whole Grains: Fiber and nutrients from whole grains like quinoa, brown rice, and oats can help reduce inflammation.

Spices and Herbs: The anti-inflammatory properties of turmeric, ginger, garlic, cinnamon, and other spices can be easily incorporated into dishes.

Balancing Your Plate for Anti-Inflammation Achieving a balanced intake of these foods is an important part of the anti-inflammatory diet. The objective is not to eliminate all potentially inflammatory foods; rather, it is to develop a nutritional strategy that is both balanced and long-lasting. Some suggestions:

Including a Variety: Differentiate your eating regimen with a great many brilliant organic products, vegetables, lean proteins, and entire grains.

Pick Sound Fats: Reduce saturated and trans fats while maximizing sources of healthy fats like avocados, olive oil, and fatty fish.

Cooking mindfully: Try experimenting with healthy oil-based cooking methods like steaming, roasting, and sautéing to preserve flavors and nutrients.

Segment Control: Because overeating, even of healthy foods, can contribute to inflammation, pay attention to portion sizes.

Women can tailor their diets to boost anti-inflammatory responses in their bodies by understanding the science behind these dietary choices. I will look at practical strategies and delicious recipes that use these anti-inflammatory foods in the coming chapters. This will help women use their diet to support their overall health and vitality.

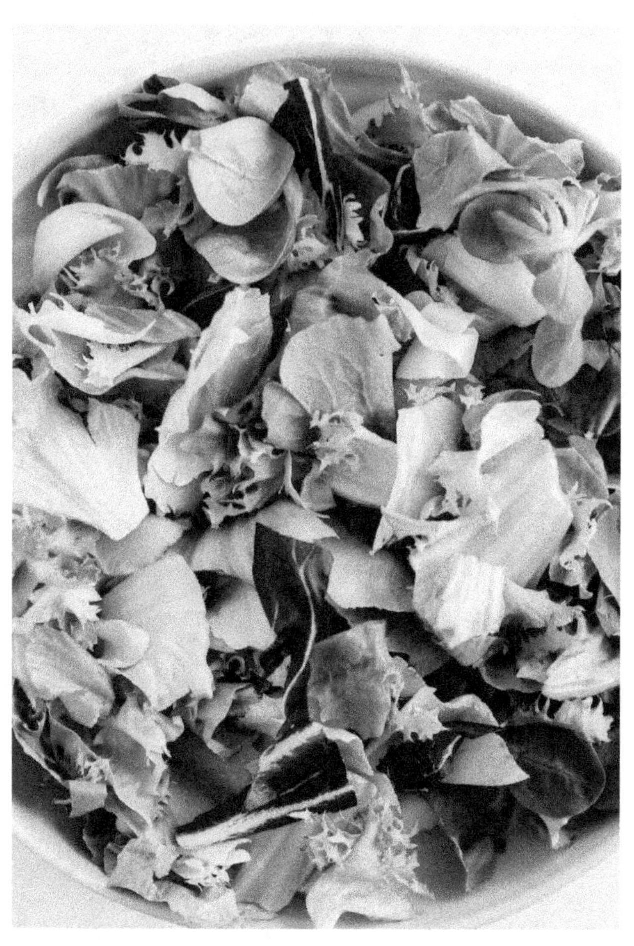

Chapter 3: Getting Started on Your Anti-Inflammatory Journey

To set out on any journey, you need to have the right mindset, be prepared, and know where to go. Your quest for a comprehensive, women-specific anti-inflammatory diet is not unusual. In this chapter, I will give you the fundamental devices, methodologies, and a bit by bit guide to start your extraordinary calming venture.

Consider this chapter as your launchpad, the point of departure from which you will begin your journey toward vibrant health and well-being. This chapter will set the stage for the practical, actionable advice and delicious recipes that await you in the subsequent chapters, whether you are a newcomer to the world of anti-inflammatory living or seeking to deepen your understanding and commitment.

Thus, I should make a plunge, begin, and take those significant first walks toward a better, more lively you through the total mitigating diet for women.

Assessing Your Current Diet and Lifestyle Setting Realistic Goals

The first step in starting your anti-inflammatory journey is to honestly evaluate your current situation. This step is critical as it establishes the groundwork for significant and practical changes in your eating routine and way of life. I will walk you through the steps of self-evaluation and goal setting in this section, assisting you in creating a clear path forward for your transformation.

Reviewing Your Existing Diet and Way of Life Before you can make a plan for the future, it's important to know where you started. Here are a few vital perspectives to consider as you evaluate your ongoing eating routine and way of life:

Eating Habits: Consider the meals and snacks you typically consume each day. What foods do you typically consume? Are there any particular patterns or dietary practices that stand out, whether they are beneficial or may be inflammatory?

Factors in Your Life: Past eating routine, think about your way of life decisions. How active are you physically? Do you have strategies for managing stress? Are there any habits that could be harming your health, like smoking or drinking too much alcohol?

Wellbeing and Prosperity: Assess your overall health and well-being for a moment. Are there any current ailments or side effects of irritation that you're presently managing? How would you feel on an everyday premise?

Putting forth Sensible Objectives

With an unmistakable comprehension of where you presently stand, the following stage is to lay out sensible and feasible objectives for your calming process. Setting goals gives you direction and drives you to keep going when you make changes. Consider this approach:

Explicit and Quantifiable: Your objectives ought to be precise and measurable. Specific goals, such as "consume at least five servings of vegetables daily," are preferable to vague ones like "eat healthier."

Realistic and realizable: Make goals that you can achieve given your current situation. While it's admirable to set lofty goals, they should also be attainable in the long run.

Time-Bound: Set a timetable for achieving your objectives. A sense of urgency and accountability are brought about by this. For instance, set a goal to be accomplished in three months or less.

Gradual Advancement: Keep in mind that change takes time to occur. You might want to think about starting with smaller, more manageable goals and gradually increasing your ambitions as you gain confidence and momentum.

Examples of Anti-Inflammatory Objectives To get you started, here are some examples of anti-inflammatory objectives to think about:

Increase Your Vegetarian Diet: Try to include one more serving of vegetables in each meal every day.

Hydration: To stay hydrated, make sure you drink at least eight glasses of water every day.

Getting Moving: At least three times per week, commit to 30 minutes of moderate exercise, such as brisk walking or yoga.

Careful Eating: Savor each bite and pay attention to your body's signals of hunger and fullness to practice mindful eating.

Stress Reduction: Spend ten minutes a day journaling, doing deep breathing exercises, or practicing meditation to reduce stress.

Cut back on processed foods and sugar: Replace sugary snacks and processed foods with whole, unprocessed options as you gradually reduce your intake.

You are creating a road map for your anti-inflammatory journey by setting these or similar goals that are tailored to your particular circumstances. Keep in mind that progress is a journey rather than a destination, and that each step you take forward brings you closer to becoming a happier, healthier version of yourself. I will provide you with useful strategies, delicious recipes, and useful resources in the following chapters to support your objectives and help you succeed on your anti-inflammatory path for women's health.

Creating a Supportive Environment

Creating a supportive environment can have a significant impact on your success and overall well-being as you begin your anti-inflammatory journey. In this segment, I'll investigate the significance of your environmental factors, connections, and outlook in keeping a solid and calming way of life customized for ladies.

The Power of Your Environment Your physical environment has a significant impact on the choices and habits you make every day. This is the way you can make your current circumstance helpful for a mitigating way of life:

Remodeling the Kitchen: Begin in the core of your home — the kitchen. In your pantry and refrigerator, get rid of processed foods, sugary snacks, and foods that cause inflammation. Whole grains, lean proteins, fresh produce, and anti-inflammatory ingredients are better alternatives.

Preparing a Meal: Commit time to dinner readiness. It will be easier for you to adhere to your dietary goals during busy days if you plan and prepare anti-inflammatory meals in advance.

Perceivability Matters: Keep solid tidbits like new natural products or unsalted nuts noticeable and open. This can check undesirable desires and advance better decisions.

Social Support Having a network of people who support you can completely transform your anti-inflammatory journey. How to make the most of social connections is as follows:

Discuss Your Objectives: Discuss your calming objectives with loved ones. They might even accompany you on your journey and offer support.

Track down Similar People group: Look for anti-inflammatory lifestyle groups in your area or online. Advice, motivation, and a sense of community can all be gained from participating in these communities.

Consider the Influence of Others: Be aware that social gatherings and peer pressure can sometimes challenge your dietary choices, even though sharing your goals is beneficial. Learn how to gracefully decline foods that don't support your objectives.

A Positive Outlook

Your outlook is a useful asset in your calming process. Practice cultivating a growth-oriented and upbeat mentality in the following ways:

Self-Empathy: Be caring and pardoning yourself. Recognize that setbacks do occur but do not define your journey.

Spotlight on Progress, Not Flawlessness: Go for the gold, flawlessness. Consistent, small adjustments are frequently more long-lasting and effective than complete overhauls.

Appreciation: Become more grateful. Even if they seem insignificant, acknowledge the positive aspects of your journey and the progress you're making.

Eating Mindfully: Adopt mindful eating habits. Relish each nibble, pay attention to your body's yearning and completion signals, and encourage a solid relationship with food.

Getting In a good position

By establishing a strong climate, sustaining social associations, and embracing a positive mentality, you're placing yourself in a good position on your calming process. Recollect that this excursion isn't about hardship yet about feeding your body and improving your general prosperity. I will provide you with helpful hints, delectable recipes, and direction in the following chapters to make sure you have everything you need to succeed on your way to a comprehensive anti-inflammatory diet designed specifically for women's health.

Chapter 4: Anti-Inflammatory Foods for Women

In this chapter, I will dig into the core of your mitigating venture — the food sources that can support and enable ladies to flourish. You'll find a different exhibit of scrumptious and wellbeing improving decisions that can assist with combatting constant irritation, support ladies' interesting nourishing necessities, and make ready for lively wellbeing.

Consider this chapter your culinary journey as I explore the world of women-specific anti-inflammatory foods. I'll reveal the science behind these food varieties, their significant effect on prosperity, and give down to earth direction on the most proficient method to integrate them into your day to day dinners. So, put on an apron, sharpen your knives, and get ready to go on a culinary adventure that will change your health and vitality from the inside out.

The Power of Whole Grains

Entire grains are nourishing forces to be reckoned with that can be a foundation of your calming diet custom fitted for ladies. Numerous health benefits are provided by these nutrient-dense foods, including a reduction in chronic inflammation. In this segment, I'll investigate why entire grains are an imperative part of your calming eating plan and how to make them a delectable piece of your day to day feasts.

What Are Entire Grains?

Entire grains will be grains that contain every one of the three pieces of the grain bit: the grain, microorganism, and endosperm. They keep all of their nutrients, fiber, and phytochemicals in this intact structure. Normal entire grains include:

Oats
Quinoa
Earthy colored rice
Grain
Buckwheat
Entire wheat
Millet
Farro
Amaranth
Triticale
The Calming Advantages of Entire Grains

Entire grains offer a large number of medical advantages, and their job in decreasing ongoing irritation is huge:

Fiber: Entire grains are wealthy in dietary fiber, especially dissolvable fiber. Fiber has calming properties and can assist with controlling glucose levels, which is pivotal for overseeing aggravation.

Antioxidants: Antioxidants found in whole grains reduce oxidative stress and inflammation. Vitamins, minerals, and phytochemicals like lignans are among these antioxidants.

Gut Well-Being: Fiber in entire grains upholds a solid stomach microbiome, which is progressively perceived for its job in irritation guidelines and generally wellbeing.

Managing Blood Sugar: Compared to refined grains, whole grains have a lower glycemic index, which means they help maintain blood sugar levels. This can diminish the gamble of irritation related with insulin obstruction. Including Whole Grains in Your Diet It's easier than you think to include whole grains in your diet on a regular basis. Here are a few useful ways to integrate them into your feasts:

Mealtime: A nourishing breakfast bowl made of whole grain oats or quinoa serves as the foundation. For a filling meal, drizzle honey on top of nuts, fruits, and vegetables.

Lunch: Grain bowls, salads, and wraps for lunchtime should be made with brown rice or quinoa in place of white rice. Your meal will benefit from the anti-inflammatory power and nutty flavor of these whole grains.

Supper: Try different things with various entire grains like farro, grain, or millet in your soups, stews, or grain side dishes. They can give surface and profundity to your night feasts.

Foods: For a healthy and filling snack, try air-popped popcorn, whole grain granola, or whole grain crackers.

Entire Grains for Ladies' Wellbeing

For women, entire grains offer extra advantages. They give fundamental supplements like iron, magnesium, and B nutrients, which are particularly significant for women' wellbeing. Magnesium supports bone health and relieves PMS symptoms, and B vitamins contribute to energy metabolism. Iron is essential for preventing anemia.

You can nourish your body with a wide range of nutrients while also reducing inflammation by embracing the power of whole grains. You'll be well on your way to a happier, healthier you as you discover delicious ways to include whole grains in your anti-inflammatory diet. In the parts ahead, I'll proceed with our excursion through the universe of mitigating food varieties custom fitted for ladies' special healthful necessities.

Vibrant Fruits and Vegetables

Leafy foods are the stars of your mitigating diet customized for ladies. In addition to adding color to your plate, these nutrient-dense, colorful foods offer a plethora of health benefits, including a reduction in chronic inflammation. In this section, I'll talk about the reasons why fruits and vegetables are so important to your anti-inflammatory diet and how to make them taste good and be a big part of your meals every day.

The Powerhouses of Nutrition: Leafy foods

Leafy foods are overflowing with fundamental supplements and bioactive mixtures that advance by and large wellbeing and prosperity. They are essential for an anti-inflammatory diet for the following reasons:

Cancer prevention agents: Leafy foods are plentiful in cancer prevention agents, including nutrients C and E, beta-carotene, and different phytochemicals. These antioxidants reduce body inflammation and combat oxidative stress.

Fiber: They are excellent sources of dietary fiber, particularly soluble fiber, which helps maintain a healthy gut microbiome and regulate blood sugar levels, two crucial aspects of managing inflammation.

Minerals and Vitamins: The immune system, bone health, and general vitality are all aided by a variety of vitamins and minerals found in fruits and vegetables. For instance, potassium, which is found in spinach and bananas, helps control blood pressure.

Keeping hydrated: The high water content of many fruits and vegetables aids in hydration, which is essential for overall health and reduces inflammation.

The Anti-Inflammatory Properties of Fruits and Vegetables Eating a wide variety of fruits and vegetables has the potential to have significant anti-inflammatory effects. A few explicit advantages include:

Decreasing Oxidative Pressure: Fruits and vegetables' antioxidants neutralize harmful free radicals, lowering oxidative stress and inflammation.

Reducing Markers of Inflammation: Lower levels of inflammatory markers like C-reactive protein (CRP) and interleukin-6 (IL-6) have been linked to regular consumption of these foods.

Promoting a Healthy Gut: Fruits and vegetables' fiber helps maintain a healthy and anti-inflammatory gut microbiome by providing food for beneficial gut bacteria.

Weight The executives: These foods can help you lose weight because they are usually low in calories and high in fiber, which makes you feel fuller for longer.

2.3 Including Fruits and Vegetables in Your Diet It's fun and doable to include fruits and vegetables in your diet on a regular basis. The following are some helpful hints for including them in your meals:

Variety is important: Try to include a wide range of colorful vegetables and fruits. Vitamins, minerals, and phytochemicals are unique to each color. Consider the rainbow on your plate.

Nibbling: For a healthy and filling snack, try a handful of berries, vegetable sticks with hummus, or fresh fruit.

Drinks: Mix products of the soil greens into smoothies for a reviving and supplement pressed breakfast or tidbit.

Servings of mixed greens: Make lively plates of mixed greens with a blend of vegetables, organic products, nuts, and lean proteins. For a variety of flavors, try different toppings and dressings.

Making Food: Add vegetables to stir-fries, soups, stews, and pasta dishes to include them in your main courses.

The Benefits of Fruits and Vegetables for Women's Health For women, the advantages of fruits and vegetables include supporting particular health requirements. For instance, vitamin C-rich foods like strawberries and citrus fruits can increase iron absorption, which is important for pregnant women. Folate, which is found in citrus fruits and leafy greens, is important for reproductive health, especially during pregnancy.

In addition to reducing inflammation, incorporating vibrant fruits and vegetables into your anti-inflammatory diet provides your body with a treasure trove of essential nutrients. You'll be on your way to a happier, healthier you as you discover the delicious ways to incorporate these foods into your daily diet. I will continue my investigation of anti-inflammatory foods tailored to women's specific nutritional requirements in the following chapters.

Lean Proteins and Healthy Fats

Healthy fats and lean proteins are the essential orchestrators in your anti-inflammatory diet for women. In addition to providing flavor and satiety, these macronutrients have unique health benefits, including reducing chronic inflammation. I'll explore about the importance of lean proteins and healthy fats to your anti-inflammatory diet and how to incorporate them into your daily meals in this section.

The Importance of Lean Proteins Lean proteins are good sources of essential amino acids, which your body needs to build and repair tissues and other structures. Here's the reason they are critical for a calming diet:

Strength Training: Lean proteins support muscle health, which is necessary for metabolic health and overall well-being.

Fullness: Protein-rich food sources assist you with feeling more full for longer, lessening the compulsion to nibble on provocative food sources.

Glucose Guideline: Protein can assist with settling glucose levels, diminishing irritation related to insulin obstruction.

Good Fats: Unsaturated fats, which are essential to an anti-inflammatory diet and provide numerous health benefits, are healthy fats. Here's the reason they're fundamental:

Mitigating Properties: Sound fats, particularly omega-3 unsaturated fats tracked down in greasy fish, flaxseeds, and pecans, have powerful mitigating properties.

Heart Wellbeing: By promoting healthy blood vessel function and lowering cholesterol levels, these fats can improve heart health.

Supplement Retention: Fruits and vegetables' phytonutrients and fat-soluble vitamins (A, D, E, and K) are better absorbed by healthy fats.

Mind Wellbeing: Omega-3 unsaturated fats are indispensable for mind wellbeing and may assist with decreasing the gamble of mental degradation.

Including Lean Proteins and Healthy Fats in Your Diet Eating meals that include lean proteins and healthy fats can be delicious and filling. The following are some helpful hints for including them in your diet:

High-Fat Proteins:

Decide on skinless poultry, lean cuts of hamburger or pork, tofu, tempeh, vegetables, and fish like salmon and trout.
Include quinoa, beans, lentils, chickpeas, and other plant-based protein sources in your diet.
Good Fats:

Regularly consume fatty fish like salmon, mackerel, and sardines.
Salads and snacks can benefit from the addition of olive oil, nuts, seeds, and avocados.
For a satisfying and nutritious pick-me-up, munch on a few nuts.
Fitting for Ladies' Wellbeing.

For ladies, lean proteins and solid fats are fundamental for keeping up with hormonal equilibrium, particularly during different life stages like feminine cycle, pregnancy, and menopause. Your body will have the amino acids it needs to make hormones if you eat enough protein, and healthy fats help your body absorb fat-soluble vitamins that are important for good reproductive health.

By embracing lean proteins and sound fats in your calming diet, you're feeding your body with fundamental supplements and lessening irritation. As you investigate the delectable ways of integrating these macronutrients into your everyday dinners, you'll be headed to a better, more energetic you. In the parts ahead, I'll proceed with our investigation of mitigating food varieties custom-made for ladies' extraordinary dietary requirements.

Superfoods for Women's Health

Superfoods are the nutritional powerhouses of nature because they provide a concentrated supply of phytochemicals, antioxidants, vitamins, minerals, and other nutrients that can have a significant impact on women's health. In this part, I'll dig into some noteworthy superfoods that merit a noticeable spot in your calming diet customized for ladies. These food varieties can assist with combatting irritation, support hormonal equilibrium, and improve generally speaking prosperity.

Fruit: Berries, such as blueberries, strawberries, raspberries, and blackberries, are packed with phytochemicals and antioxidants, making them potent women's anti-inflammatory superfoods:

Cell reinforcement Power: Berries are rich in anthocyanins and flavonoids, strong cell reinforcements that battle oxidative pressure and irritation.

Heart Wellbeing: Standard utilization of berries has been connected to work on cardiovascular wellbeing, including lower pulse and diminished risk factors for coronary illness.

Mental Well-Being: The cell reinforcements in berries might uphold mental capability and decrease the gamble old enough related mental degradation.

 Skin Wellbeing: The nutrients and cell reinforcements in berries can advance sound, shining skin.

Green Vegetables: Supplement Thick and Mitigating

Salad greens like spinach, kale, Swiss chard, and collard greens are supplement pressed superfoods that offer a variety of medical advantages for women.

Plentiful in Nutrients: Vitamins A, C, and K, as well as essential minerals like iron and calcium, are abundant in leafy greens.

Calming Properties: They contain phytonutrients that assist with diminishing aggravation and backing generally wellbeing.

Bone Condition: Leafy greens contain both calcium and vitamin K, which are necessary for maintaining healthy bones.

Folate for women: Folate, which can be found in leafy greens, is important for pregnant women because it helps the fetus grow during pregnancy.

Crunchy Fish: Omega-3 Rich for Mind and Heart Wellbeing

Greasy fish like salmon, mackerel, and sardines are superfoods overflowing with omega-3 unsaturated fats, offering special advantages for ladies:

Advantages of Omega-3: Fatty fish's omega-3 fatty acids are beneficial to heart and brain health and have anti-inflammatory properties.

Hormonal Equilibrium: Omega-3s may support hormonal balance and alleviate PMS symptoms.

Thinking Ability: Standard utilization of greasy fish has been connected to working on mental capability and diminished hazard of mental degradation in women.

Skin and hair: Fatty fish's omega-3 fatty acids have been shown to improve hair luster and skin health.

Turmeric: The Brilliant Zest

Turmeric, a dazzling yellow zest, contains curcumin, a compound with intense calming and cell reinforcement properties:

Effects on inflammation: Curcumin has been read up for its capacity to lessen irritation, making it a significant expansion to a mitigating diet.

Joint Wellbeing: Turmeric may alleviate joint stiffness and pain, two common issues that women face as they get older.

Balance of Hormones: Curcumin may help women maintain their hormonal balance, according to some research.

The Digestive System: Turmeric can help with stomach related wellbeing by diminishing side effects of heartburn and advancing stomach wellbeing.

Flaxseeds: Omega-3 Fatty Acids and Fiber Flax Seeds are a nutrient powerhouse high in omega-3 fatty acids, fiber, and lignans. They have a number of advantages for women, including the following:

Omega-3 Fats: Omega-3 fatty acids, which are beneficial to heart and brain health, can be found in flaxseeds, a plant-based source.

Hormonal Wellbeing: Flaxseeds' lignans may aid in hormone balance and lower the risk of hormone-related cancers.

Stomach related Consistency: Flaxseeds' fiber aids in gut health and encourages regular bowel movements.

Skin and hair: Omega-3 fatty acids found in flaxseeds support healthy hair and skin.

Integrating Superfoods into Your Eating regimen

Consolidating superfoods into your mitigating diet is both pleasant and fulfilling. Here are a few down to earth ways to incorporate them into your dinners:

Berry Smoothies: Mix berries with salad greens and Greek yogurt for a supplement pressed morning smoothie.

Dinners with Salmon: Appreciate greasy fish like salmon barbecued or heated with a side of salad greens and a turmeric-based sauce.

Turmeric Tea: As a calming and anti-inflammatory beverage, sip turmeric tea.

Flaxseed Breakfast: Distribute the ground flaxseeds.

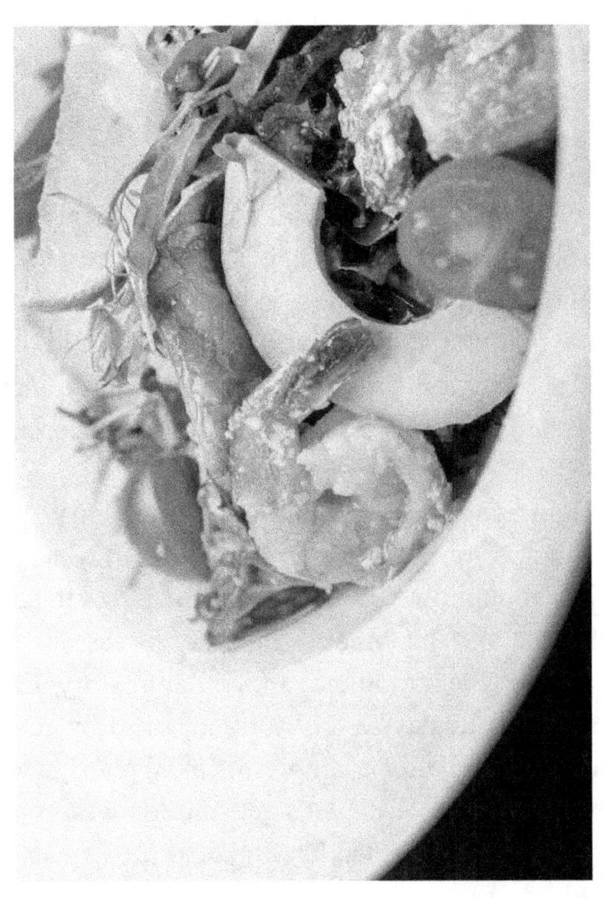

Chapter 5: Anti-Inflammatory Meal Planning

The art of turning your anti-inflammatory diet goals into everyday choices is called meal planning. In this chapter, I'll plunge into the fundamental standards of feast arranging custom-made for ladies. This chapter will provide you with the knowledge and tools to prepare healthy, anti-inflammatory meals that support your health and well-being, regardless of your cooking experience.

In the fight against chronic inflammation, consider meal planning to be your secret weapon. It's about what you eat as well as about how you structure your feasts to advance nourishment and happiness. In order to assist you in incorporating the complete anti-inflammatory diet for women into your day-to-day routine, meal by meal, I'll look at strategies, offer examples of meal plans, and offer helpful advice. Therefore, let's get started on this culinary journey toward greater vitality and health.

Building Balanced Meals

Women-specific anti-inflammatory diet centers on creating healthy meals. These well-planned meals provide necessary nutrients, keep you full, and aid in the fight against chronic inflammation. In this section, I'll investigate the critical parts of adjusted feasts and give viable direction on the most proficient method to make them.

The Elements of a Well-Balanced Meal A well-balanced meal typically includes the following elements:

Lean Protein: Protein is necessary for the immune system, muscle health, and overall vitality. Pick lean wellsprings of protein like poultry, fish, tofu, vegetables, or lean cuts of meat.

Whole Grains: Complex carbohydrates, dietary fiber, vitamins, and minerals are found in whole grains. Integrate choices like earthy colored rice, quinoa, entire wheat pasta, or oats.

Plenty of Greens: A wide variety of vitamins, minerals, antioxidants, and fiber can be found in vegetables. Try to eat half of your plate of colorful, non-starchy vegetables like broccoli, peppers, carrots, and leafy greens.

Good Fats: Olive oil, avocados, nuts, and seeds are all good sources of healthy fat. These fats support heart and mind wellbeing and improve the kind of your dishes.

Additional Superfoods: To increase the nutritional value of your meals and provide specific health benefits, include superfoods like turmeric, berries, and leafy greens.

Creating Healthy Breakfasts Because your breakfast sets the tone for the rest of your day, it's important to start with a healthy meal:

Options High in Protein: Consider Greek yogurt, curds, or fried eggs as wellsprings of protein.

Grains as a Whole: Oatmeal, whole grain toast, and whole grain cereal are all examples of whole grain options.

Vegetables or Fruits: Integrate natural products like berries or cut bananas, or add vegetables to omelets or breakfast bowls.

Good Fats: Sprinkle nuts or seeds on your yogurt or shower olive oil over your avocado toast.

Creating Well-Balanced Lunches Your lunch should give you energy all day long:

Lean Meat: Utilize barbecued chicken, tofu, or beans as a protein base for servings of mixed greens, wraps, or grain bowls.

Grains as a Whole: Choose brown rice, whole grain bread, or quinoa for your meal's base.

Plenty of Greens: Load your lunch with various bright vegetables for nutrients and fiber.

Good Fats: Slices of avocado, a drizzle of olive oil, or a few nuts can all be added.

Structure Adjusted Meals

Supper is a chance to loosen up and sustain your body:

Lean Protein: Take pleasure in fish, lean meat cuts, and plant-based proteins like lentils.

Grains as a Whole: Serve whole grains for dinner, such as quinoa, farro, or whole wheat pasta.

Plentiful Vegetables: Serve plenty of vegetables on a well-balanced plate as a side dish or as part of the main dish.

Sound Fats: A side of roasted nuts, olive oil, or seeds can all add flavor and nutrients to your dish.

Snacks and Mini-Meals When necessary, include healthy snacks and mini-meals:

Foodstuffs: Eat hummus with vegetables, Greek yogurt, or a hard-boiled egg for a snack.

Fiber: Pick fiber-rich choices like entire natural products, entire grain saltines, or a little plate of mixed greens.

Control of portions: In order to maintain a healthy weight and avoid overeating, pay attention to portion sizes.

Hydration Is Important Include hydration in your balanced meal plan. You can support your overall health and stay hydrated by drinking water, herbal teas, and water infused with citrus or berry slices.

Making adjusted feasts is a central part of your mitigating diet. You can give your body the nutrients it needs to thrive and effectively fight inflammation by including superfoods, whole grains, plenty of vegetables, healthy fats, and lean proteins in your diet. In the parts ahead, I'll proceed with our investigation of dinner arranging, giving functional direction and test feast plans custom-made to your mitigating venture.

Weekly Meal Planning Tips

If you want to successfully incorporate an anti-inflammatory diet into your life, the key is to plan your meals well. Week by week dinner arranging permits you to save time, diminish food squander, and guarantee that you have adjusted and nutritious feasts prepared consistently. In this part, I'll investigate a few fundamental tips and methodologies to assist you with turning into an expert at week by week dinner arranging, custom fitted for ladies' exceptional healthful necessities.

Set Specific Objectives Before beginning your weekly meal planning, clearly define your anti-inflammatory diet's objectives. Take into account your dietary preferences, health objectives, and any dietary requirements you may have. Having an unmistakable vision of what you need to accomplish will direct your dinner arranging choices.

Make a Week by week Timetable

Plan a week by week feast, arranging a plan that suits your way of life. Consider your work hours, family responsibilities, and any friendly exercises. Having an organized arrangement will make it simpler to designate time for feast readiness and shopping for food.

Arrangement Adjusted Dinners

Allude back to the standards of adjusted dinners examined before in this section. Make sure that every meal contains healthy fats, lean proteins, whole grains, a lot of vegetables, and maybe even superfoods. If you want to give your body a wide range of nutrients, variety is essential.

Take into consideration batch cooking. In batch cooking, more meals are made at once and then divided into smaller portions for later consumption. This is a great way to save time. Consider committing a day every week to bunch cook staples like grains, proteins, and sauces that can be utilized in different dishes.

Hug Extras

Try not to neglect the force of extras. Plan dinners that can be effectively warmed or reused into new dishes. On busy days when you don't have much time to prepare meals, leftovers can be a lifesaver.

Make a Comprehensive Shopping List Based on Your Weekly Meal Plan Before You Go to the Grocery Store This list not only helps you avoid making impulsive purchases that might not be in line with your anti-inflammatory objectives, but it also ensures that you have all of the ingredients you need.

Be Smart When grocery shopping, stick to the store's perimeters, which are typically where you'll find fresh produce, lean proteins, and whole grains. Be aware of perusing food names to keep away from exceptionally handled and fiery food varieties.

Use Innovation for Your Potential benefit

Various feast arranging applications and sites can improve on the interaction. You can often use these tools to input your dietary preferences, make shopping lists, and even get ideas for recipes based on what you already have on hand.

Mix and Match Ingredients In order to save money and reduce waste, choose recipes that share their components. For instance, in the event that you purchase a heap of new basil for a pesto pasta dish, think about involving the excess basil in servings of mixed greens or sandwiches later in the week.

Be adaptable While a well-organized meal plan is necessary, adaptability is just as important. Life can be erratic, and in some cases plans change. Don't be too hard on yourself if things don't go exactly as planned, and be open to making any necessary adjustments to your meal plan.

Prepare and Pack Ahead If you have a busy schedule, it's best to prepare meals and snacks in advance. Make it simple to grab a nourishing option while on the go by investing in handy containers for portioning and storing your meals.

Survey and Reflect

Toward the week's end, pause for a minute to survey your dinner plan's prosperity. Consider what functioned admirably and what could be moved along. Use this feedback to improve your meal planning efforts in the future.

By executing these week by week dinner arranging tips, you'll smooth out your calming diet excursion and put yourself in a good position. Preparing guarantees that you have the right food varieties available, diminishes the compulsion to pursue less sound decisions, and eventually assists you with accomplishing your wellbeing and health objectives as a feature of the total calming diet for women.

Sample Meal Plans for Different Lifestyles and Dietary Preferences

Feast arranging can be adaptable and customized to different ways of life and dietary inclinations. In order to ensure that you can tailor the anti-inflammatory diet to your specific requirements, I have provided sample meal plans for a variety of scenarios in this section. These sample meal plans provide direction and motivation to incorporate anti-inflammatory eating into your daily life, regardless of whether you are a vegetarian, a professional with a busy schedule, or have particular dietary requirements.

A Preliminary Meal Plan: Breakfast with an Omnivore Balance: whole grain toast, scrambled eggs with tomatoes, spinach, and berries, and a side of berries.
Snack: Greek yogurt with honey and almonds.
Lunch: Mixed greens, quinoa, and a balsamic vinaigrette dressing make up this grilled chicken salad.
Snack: Cut cucumber and carrot sticks with hummus.
Dinner: Heated salmon with lemon and dill, earthy colored rice, steamed broccoli, and a little side plate of mixed greens.
Second Sample Meal Plan: Breakfast with Vegetarian Delights: Almond milk, chia seeds, and a topping of mixed berries are added to overnight oats.

Snack: A modest bunch of blended nuts and dried natural products.

Lunch: Stir-fry vegetables and chickpeas with quinoa.

Snack: Flaxseeds and honey are drizzled over Greek yogurt.

Dinner: Curry of lentils and roasted vegetables served with brown rice and sautéed spinach on the side.

An Example of a Meal Plan: Breakfast that is gluten-free and vegan: Bowl of vegan smoothies topped with sliced almonds and berries, spinach, banana, and almond milk.

Snack: sliced avocado served with a pinch of sea salt on gluten-free rice cakes.

Lunch: Corn, black beans, roasted sweet potatoes, and a cilantro-lime dressing make up this quinoa salad.

Snack: A little bowl of blended organic product salad.

Dinner: Stew made with vegan lentils, vegetables, and gluten-free quinoa.

An Example of a Meal Plan: Professional Breakfast on the Go: Smoothie that you can grab and go with spinach, protein powder, almond milk, and some almond butter.

Snack: Hummus and vegetable sticks cut in advance

Lunch: Pre-made salad container with layers of greens, chickpeas, cherry tomatoes, and a vinaigrette dressing.

Snack: a piece of fruit or a protein bar.

Dinner: Prepared chicken bosom with steamed asparagus and a quinoa pilaf.

Example Dinner Plan 5: Breakfast in Paradise for Pescatarians: Smoked salmon and avocado on entire grain toast, finished off with a poached egg.

Snack: pineapple chunks in cottage cheese.

Lunch: Mixed greens, olives, cherry tomatoes, and a lemon-tahini dressing make up this tuna salad.

Snack: A modest bunch of cherry tomatoes and cucumber cuts.

Dinner: Skewers of grilled shrimp, quinoa salad, and roasted Brussels sprouts.

The anti-inflammatory diet's adaptability to various lifestyles and dietary preferences is demonstrated by these sample meal plans. Use them as a starting point, and you can change them to better meet your requirements and preferences. Keep in mind that meal planning is a fluid process that you can modify as your preferences and schedule shift. As a component of the complete anti-inflammatory diet for women, the objective is to develop a sustainable and pleasurable eating regimen that is beneficial to your health and well-being.

Chapter 6: Cooking and Meal Preparation

The kitchen is the center of your anti-inflammatory journey. In this part, I'll plunge into the craftsmanship and study of preparing and feast arrangement custom-made for the total mitigating diet for ladies. Cooking is about more than just feeding your body; It's a fun and creative way to take charge of your health and enjoy the flavors of healthy, anti-inflammatory ingredients.

This section will direct you through fundamental cooking procedures, dinner arrangement systems, and the significance of careful cooking. Whether you're a seasoned cook or just starting out, you'll find helpful hints and suggestions to incorporate anti-inflammatory cooking into your daily routine. Therefore, don your apron, sharpen your knives, and join me on this culinary adventure.

Time-Saving Kitchen Tools

Effectiveness in the kitchen is fundamental, particularly while following a mitigating diet customized for women. Tools for the kitchen that save time can make cooking easier and more enjoyable while also saving you time. I'll look at a few kitchen gadgets and appliances that can help you save time while making healthy, anti-inflammatory meals in this section.

Food Processor

A food processor is a flexible device that can cleave, cut, dice, shred, and puree various fixings rapidly. It is especially useful for making sauces, preparing vegetables for salads, and making homemade dips like pesto or hummus.

Blender Making sauces, soups, and smoothies all require a high-quality blender. Look for one that has enough power to blend nuts, fibrous vegetables, and frozen fruits with ease. Using cashews or avocados, you can also use it to make creamy, dairy-free dressings and sauces.

Submersion Blender

A drenching blender, otherwise called a stick blender, is a minimized and effective device for mixing soups and sauces straightforwardly in the pot. It wipes out the need to move hot fluids to a conventional blender, saving both time and dishes.

Sluggish Cooker or Stewing pot

A sluggish cooker is an efficient marvel for occupied people. With negligible planning in the first part of the day, you can get back to a blistering, prepared feast at night. It can be used to make hearty stews, braised dishes, and even breakfast oatmeal.

Pressure Cooker or Instant Pot Using an electric pressure cooker or Instant Pot can significantly shorten the time it takes to cook grains, beans, and meat that is tougher. A flexible device joins different cooking strategies, for example, pressure cooking, slow cooking, and sauteing, in one machine.

Mandoline Slicer Using a mandoline slicer, you can cut fruits and vegetables consistently and precisely. It's ideal for making slight cuts for servings of mixed greens, gratins, and trims. When slicing, make sure to use the safety guard to protect your hands.

Vegetable Spiralizer Using a spiralizer, you can make vegetable noodles out of carrots, sweet potatoes, zucchini, and other vegetables. It's a great way to add variety to your meals without having to use traditional pasta.

Plate of mixed greens Spinner

A plate of mixed greens spinner makes washing and drying salad greens and spices a breeze. Greens that are dried don't need to be patted dry with paper towels, so they stay fresher for longer.

Spice Stripper

This helpful contraption rapidly eliminates leaves from spices like kale, thyme, and rosemary. It makes it easier to add fresh herbs to your dishes without having to pick each leaf individually.

Rice Cooker With little effort, a rice cooker guarantees perfectly cooked grains every time. Some models also have a steaming function that lets you cook rice while you prepare vegetables.

Air Fryer
An air fryer cooks food without using much oil by using hot air to crisp it up. It's incredible for accomplishing a fresh surface on food varieties like yam fries, chicken wings, or vegetable chips while lessening the general fat substance.

Nut Milk Bag A nut milk bag is a useful tool for making smooth, pulp-free nut milk and straining homemade broths and juices.

Kitchen Timer Keeping track of cooking times with a dependable kitchen timer will ensure that your meals do not overcook or undercook. Multiple alarms on many kitchen timers make it simple to manage multiple dishes at once.

Food Scale Using a food scale allows you to accurately measure the proportions of ingredients in recipes. It is especially useful for portion control and baking.

When it comes to anti-inflammatory cooking, investing in these time-saving kitchen tools can make a big difference. By diminishing planning time and working on complex errands, these contraptions permit you to zero in on making delectable and nutritious feasts that help your wellbeing as a component of the total mitigating diet for women.

Batch Cooking and Meal Prep Strategies

Effective feast readiness is a unique advantage while following a mitigating diet custom fitted for women. Meal prep and batch cooking techniques not only save you time but also ensure that you always have healthy, anti-inflammatory meals on hand. In this segment, I'll investigate the craft of clump preparing and dinner prep, giving you viable techniques to make this fundamental part of your eating regimen a consistent and charming piece of your everyday practice.

The Advantages of Group Cooking

Group cooking includes getting ready bigger amounts of food immediately and afterward partitioning it for future utilization. Here are the advantages:

Time Investment funds: Clump cooking permits you to cook once and partake in various feasts. This is particularly important on occupied days.

Less food goes to waste: It assists you with spending fixings before they turn sour, diminishing food squander.

Piece Control: Pre-distributed dinners and bites make it more straightforward to control segment estimates and abstain from gorging.

Consistency: Clump cooking guarantees that you reliably have calming feasts accessible, making it simpler to adhere to your dietary objectives.

Dinner Prep Systems

Arrange Your Dinners: Begin by making a week by week feast plan that incorporates breakfast, lunch, supper, and bites. Pick recipes that are reasonable for group cooking.

Pick Mitigating Recipes: Select recipes that line up with your mitigating diet objectives. Center around entire, natural fixings wealthy in supplements and low in added sugars and undesirable fats.

Shop Shrewd: In the wake of arranging your dinners, make a definite shopping list. This limits the possibilities of neglecting key fixings and forestall drive buys.

Preparation Materials: Start your feast prep by washing, cleaving, and dividing fixings. This can incorporate vegetables, organic products, and proteins.

Cluster Cook Staples: Spend a few hours or a day batch-cooking staples like rice, quinoa, proteins like chicken, beans, and tofu, and sauces like tomato sauce. Cook these in bigger amounts and store them in partitioned holders.

Hug Cooler Dinners: A few dishes, similar to soups, stews, and meals, freeze outstandingly well. Get ready bigger clusters, segment them into cooler safe holders, and mark them with dates for simple pivot.

Put resources into Quality Compartments: Utilize various holders in various sizes to store your prepared fixings and feasts. Settle on impenetrable, stackable holders that are microwave and dishwasher safe.

Mark and Date: Mark your compartments with the items and date of readiness to assist with association and turn.

Snacks before the meal: Segment out snacks like nuts, seeds, and cut-up vegetables in and out compartments to control thoughtless eating and settle on better decisions.

Make Feast Units: Collect dinner packs for recipes that require different parts. For example, consolidate pre-cooked proteins, grains, and vegetables in a solitary holder for simple gathering.

Be Aware of Stockpiling: Guarantee legitimate capacity conditions, like refrigeration for perishables and freezing for feasts with a more drawn out time span of usability.

Turn and Invigorate: Consume your prepared feasts inside a sensible time period to keep up with newness and supplement quality. Keep your meals fresh by rotating your batch-cooked items frequently.

Modify Parts: Consider parceling bigger bunches into individual or family-sized servings to oblige your family's requirements.

Time-Saving Tips Additional time-saving strategies include the following:

Create a Meal Preparation Timeline: Meal preparation should be prioritized on specific days or times each week. Consistency is critical to progress.

Multitasking: Utilize your time effectively by cooking numerous parts all the while, for example, broiling vegetables while setting up a sauce.

Arrangement for Extras: Cook additional servings of supper to act as lunch the following day or freeze for future feasts.

Pre-Pack Snacks: In the event that you have a bustling week's worth of work, pre-pack snacks for every day to guarantee you have a reasonable, calming feast promptly accessible.

Keep It Basic: Begin with essential dinner prep procedures, and as you become more agreeable, explore different avenues regarding more complicated recipes and methods.

By integrating cluster preparing and feast prep into your daily schedule, you'll acquire significant time and guarantee that mitigating dinners are available at whatever point you want them. Whether you're a bustling proficient, a parent with a rushed timetable, or just hoping to improve on your life, these systems are your partners in keeping a steady and wellbeing centered diet as a feature of the total calming diet for women.

Chapter 7: Delicious Anti-Inflammatory Recipes

Welcome to the culinary heart of your excursion toward better wellbeing and prosperity. In this section, I'll investigate a delicious universe of calming recipes uniquely created for women. These recipes are tied in with eating for wellbeing as well as about enjoying the kinds of feeding fixings that help your body's special necessities.

You have learned about the significance of an anti-inflammatory diet, the science behind it, and the art of meal planning and preparation in the preceding chapters. With a collection of delectable recipes that make healthy eating a delightful experience, it's time to put that knowledge into practice.

These recipes, which include vibrant salads, hearty main dishes, and mouthwatering desserts, are intended to tantalize your taste buds while also promoting optimal health. Whether you're cooking for yourself, your family, or engaging visitors, these recipes will assist you with making paramount feasts that line up with the total calming diet for women.

In this way, I should focus in, put on our covers, and leave on a tasty excursion toward better wellbeing and health through scrumptious calming cooking.

Breakfasts to Start Your Day Right

Breakfast is many times hailed as the main dinner of the day, and for good explanation. It gives the energy and supplements expected to launch your day and establishes the vibe for your dietary patterns. In this segment, I'll investigate an assortment of calming breakfast recipes custom-made for women that are nutritious as well as delightful. Your mind and body will be nourished by these recipes, which will help you get your day off to a good start.

Ingredients for the Quinoa and Berry Breakfast Bowl:

1/2 cup cooked quinoa
1/2 cup blended berries (strawberries, blueberries, raspberries)
1 tablespoon honey or maple syrup
2 tablespoons hacked nuts (almonds, pecans, or pistachios)
1/4 cup Greek yogurt (or without dairy elective)

A sprinkle of cinnamon
Directions:

In a bowl, consolidate the cooked quinoa and blended berries.
Sprinkle the top with honey or maple syrup.
Add a touch of Greek yogurt and sprinkle with hacked nuts and cinnamon.
Partake in your protein-pressed and cancer prevention agent rich breakfast bowl.
1.1.2 Avocado Toast with Poached Egg

Fixings:

1 cut of entire grain bread (or without gluten bread)
1/2 ready avocado, squashed
1 poached egg
Salt and pepper to taste
A touch of red pepper drops (discretionary)
New spices for embellish (like parsley or cilantro)
Directions:

Toast the entire grain bread until browns.
Spread the squashed avocado over the toast.
Top with an impeccably poached egg and season with salt, pepper, and red pepper drops whenever wanted.
Add fresh herbs to the dish for flavor and nutrition.
1.1.3 Spinach and Mushroom Breakfast Quesadilla

Fixings:

2 entire grain tortillas (or sans gluten tortillas)
1 cup new spinach leaves
1/2 cup cut mushrooms
2 eggs, mixed
1/4 cup destroyed cheddar (discretionary)
Salt and pepper to taste
Olive oil for cooking
Guidelines:

In a skillet, sauté the cut mushrooms and spinach in olive oil until shriveled.
Eliminate the vegetables from the skillet and put away.
In a similar skillet, scramble the eggs until cooked through.
Place a tortilla in the skillet and layer with fried eggs, sautéed vegetables, and destroyed cheddar (whenever wanted).
Top with the subsequent tortilla and cook until the two sides are brilliant and the cheddar is dissolved.
Cut into wedges and serve your flavorful and protein-pressed quesadilla.
1.1.4 Berries and Chia Seed Pudding Ingredients:

2 tablespoons chia seeds
1/2 cup almond milk (or any flavored milk)

1/2 teaspoon vanilla concentrate

1 tablespoon honey or maple syrup

1/2 cup blended berries (strawberries, blueberries, raspberries)

Directions:

In a bowl, blend the chia seeds, almond milk, vanilla concentrate, and honey or maple syrup.

Mix well and refrigerate for no less than two hours or expedite to permit the chia seeds to ingest the fluid and make a pudding-like surface.

For a nutritious and filling breakfast, top with a mix of berries.

These tasty breakfast recipes are only the start of your culinary excursion to help your wellbeing with a mitigating diet. They nourish your body with essential nutrients and energy in a flavorful and nutritious way to start your day. Partake in these morning delights as a feature of the total calming diet for ladies, and feel the advantages over the course of your day.

Energizing Lunches

The opportunity to replenish your body and maintain your energy throughout the remainder of the day is provided by lunch. I'll look at some revitalizing and anti-inflammatory lunch meals specifically geared toward women in this part. These meals are created to provide you a pleasant blend of flavors and nutrients that will leave you feeling full and invigorated.

Salad of quinoa and chickpeas

Ingredients:

cooked quinoa, 1 cup
1 cup washed and drained canned chickpeas
1 cucumber, chopped, and 1 cup cherry tomatoes
14 cup coarsely chopped red onion
14 cup chopped fresh parsley
lemon juice from one
Olive oil, two tablespoons
pepper and salt as desired
Feta cheese crumbles (optional)
Instructions:

The cooked quinoa, chickpeas, cherry tomatoes, cucumber, red onion, and fresh parsley should all be combined in a big bowl.
To make the dressing, combine the lemon juice, olive oil, salt, and pepper in a separate small bowl.
Over the salad, drizzle the dressing, and mix to blend.
For an additional flavor and creaminess boost, sprinkle some crumbled feta cheese on top if preferred.

Enjoy your quinoa and chickpea salad, which is high in fiber and protein.

2.1.2 Soup with lentils and sweet potatoes

Ingredients:

Olive oil, 1 tbsp
2 medium sweet potatoes, peeled and diced 1 medium onion, chopped 2 cloves of minced garlic
1 cup washed red lentils
Six cups of vegetable stock
1 teaspoon of cumin, ground
One-half teaspoon of ground turmeric
pepper and salt as desired
garnish with fresh cilantro
Instructions:

The oil of olives should be heated in a large pot over medium heat. When aromatic and transparent, add the minced onion and garlic.

Stir in the red lentils, cumin, turmeric, salt, and pepper along with the sweet potatoes and vegetable broth.

The sweet potatoes and lentils should be cooked through after 20 to 25 minutes of simmering after the mixture comes to a boil.

Until the soup is creamy, purée it using an immersion blender. The soup should be carefully transferred in batches to a blender and blend until smooth if you don't have an immersion blender.

Serve the soup hot with fresh cilantro on top.

2.1.3 Quinoa with Grilled Chicken Bowl

Ingredients:

cooked quinoa, 1 cup

Sliced 6 ounces of grilled chicken breast and 1 cup of mixed greens (arugula, spinach, and kale).

Half a cup of cherry tomatoes

14 cup of cucumber slices

chopped 1/4 cup red bell pepper

Goat cheese crumbles, 1/4 cup (optional)

dressing made with balsamic vinegar

Instructions:

Prepared quinoa, grilled chicken, mixed greens, cherry tomatoes, cucumbers, and red bell pepper should be arranged in a bowl.

If preferred, top with goat cheese crumbles.

Add a balsamic vinaigrette dressing drizzle.

Toss the ingredients together gently.

Enjoy a lunch bowl that is nutrient- and protein-rich.

2.1.4 Wrap with salmon and avocado

Ingredients:

a single whole-grain or gluten-free flatbread
Salmon, grilled or baked, 4 ounces
sliced avocados, half ripe
baby spinach leaves, 1/4 cup
Carrots, shredded, 14 cup
For drizzling, use Greek yogurt or tahini sauce
juice of fresh lemons
pepper and salt as desired
Instructions:

Flatten the whole-wheat dough.
In the center, arrange the salmon, slices of avocado, baby spinach, and shredded carrots.
Add a squeeze of fresh lemon juice and some Greek yogurt or tahini sauce.
To taste, add salt and pepper to the food.
To make a wrap, roll up the tortilla and tuck the sides in.
Enjoy a protein- and omega-3-rich meal by slicing in half.
These energetic lunch recipes provide you a pleasant noon pick-me-up so you can stay alert and energized the rest of the day. Use these delectable dishes as part of your anti-inflammatory diet for women and enjoy the flavors and health advantages they provide.

Nourishing Dinners

Dinner is a chance to fuel your body with a decent and mitigating dinner made only for ladies. It's likewise a chance to rest and partake in a dinner with friends and family. I'll take a gander at a couple of feasts in this space that are made to give you the sustenance and satiation you really want to unwind your day in a sound manner.

Broiled vegetables and heated salmon

Fixings:

4 salmon filets, each gauging 6 to 8 ounces
2 cups of blended vegetables, including zucchini, ringer peppers, broccoli, and carrots
Olive oil, two tablespoons
1 finely cut lemon
2 minced garlic cloves
one tablespoon of dried thyme
pepper and salt as wanted
Guidelines:

Turn on the stove to 400 °F (200 °C).
Consolidate the blended vegetables in an enormous bowl and season with salt, pepper, cleaved garlic, and olive oil.
Vegetables are fanned out on a baking skillet.
Over the vegetables, orchestrate the salmon filets.

On every salmon filet, place a cut of lemon.

Salmon ought to be prepared for 15 to 20 minutes, or until it chips promptly with a fork.

For a filling supper, serve your omega-3-rich salmon with simmered vegetables.

3.1.2 Stuffed ringer peppers with quinoa and dark beans

Fixings:

4 major, any variety chime peppers
cooked quinoa, 1 cup
1 cup washed and depleted canned dark beans
1 cup new or frozen corn pieces
Diced tomatoes, 1 cup
1/2 cup red onion, hacked
(Discretionary) 1/2 cup destroyed cheddar
1 teaspoon of cumin, ground
50 ml of stew powder
pepper and salt as wanted
embellish with new cilantro
Directions:

Set your stove's temperature to 375°F (190°C).

Eliminate the chime peppers' tops, then, at that point, scoop out the seeds and films.

Cooked quinoa, dark beans, corn, diced tomatoes, red onion, destroyed cheddar (if utilizing), ground cumin, stew powder, salt, and pepper should be generally blended in a major bowl.

Place a portion of the quinoa and dark bean blend inside each chime pepper.

Place the stuffed peppers in a baking tray and cover with foil.

Prepare the peppers for 30-35 minutes, or until they are delicate.

Prior to serving, embellish with new cilantro.

3.1.3 Tofu and Vegetable Pan fried food

Fixings:

1 cubed block of extra-firm tofu

Broccoli, ringer peppers, and snap peas make up two cups of blended veggies.

2 tablespoons of tamari (or low-sodium soy sauce for without gluten choices)

one teaspoon of sesame oil

2 minced garlic cloves

1 teaspoon ground new ginger

12 teaspoon (or more, to taste) red pepper chips

2 green onions, daintily cut Embellishment: sesame seeds

Directions:

Cut the meat into 3D squares in the wake of squeezing it to kill more dampness.

Heat the sesame oil over medium-high intensity in a major skillet or wok.

Add the red pepper pieces, ground ginger, and minced garlic. Pan sear briefly.

Cook the tofu 3D shapes, blending periodically, until sautéed and simply starting to fresh up.

Pan sear the blended vegetables for a further a few minutes.

When everything is completely covered, add the low-sodium soy sauce and stew for an extra 1-2 minutes.

Prior to serving, decorate with sesame seeds and meagerly cut green onions.

3.1.4 Vegetable and Lentil Curry

Fixings:

1 cup washed dried green or earthy colored lentils
1 diced onion, 2 minced garlic cloves
1/fourth cup curry powder
1 teaspoon of cumin, ground
One-half teaspoon of ground turmeric
1/8 teaspoon coriander powder
One 14-ounce can destroyed tomatoes
2 cups of blended veggies (cauliflower, carrots, and peas)
and 2 cups of vegetable stock
50 ml of coconut milk
pepper and salt as wanted
embellish with new cilantro

Directions:

The hacked onion and minced garlic ought to be cooked till delicate in a major pot.

Cook for 2 extra minutes subsequent to adding the curry powder, ground cumin, ground turmeric, and ground coriander.

Pour in the vegetable stock, diced tomatoes, lentils that have been washed, and blended veggies. At the point when the lentils and vegetables are cooked, stew for 20 to 25 minutes subsequent to heating to the point of boiling.

Cook for a further five minutes in the wake of adding the coconut milk.

Embellish with new cilantro and salt and pepper to taste.

Over cooked earthy colored rice or quinoa, serve your good lentil and vegetable curry.

These sound supper dishes have been made to give you a filling and wellbeing cognizant feast that advances your overall prosperity. Partaking in the flavors and wellbeing benefits these tasty recipes give to your night feasts by remembering them for your mitigating diet for women.

Satisfying Snacks and Desserts

Even in the context of an anti-inflammatory diet, sweets and snacks can help you achieve your health goals while still being delectable. This section I will look at a number of enjoyable snacks and desserts that also adhere to the fundamentals of the entire anti-inflammatory diet for women.

4.1 Nutritious Snacks

4.1.1 Banana and Nut Butter Bites

Ingredients:

cut two medium bananas
4 tablespoons of cashew, almond, or peanut butter
Chia seeds, 2 tablespoons
2 teaspoons of unsweetened coconut shreds
1/four teaspoons of cinnamon
Instructions:

Banana slices with nut butter on them.
Cinnamon, chia seeds, and coconut flakes should be added on top.
Take pleasure in these nutrient-rich nibbles as a filling snack.
Roasted chickpeas, 4.1.2

Ingredients:

One can (15 ounces) of cleaned and emptied chickpeas

Olive oil, 1 tbsp
1 teaspoon of cumin, ground
smoked paprika, 1 teaspoon
one-half teaspoon of garlic powder
Salt as desired
Instructions:

Switch on the oven to 400 degrees Celsius (200 °C).
Utilizing a paper towel, thoroughly dry the chickpeas.
Chickpeas should be mixed with salt, cumin, smoked paprika, garlic powder, and olive oil in a bowl.
On a baking sheet, distribute the chickpeas in a single layer.
Chickpeas should be roasted for 25 to 30 minutes, occasionally shaking the pan to ensure even cooking.
Before serving these protein-rich snacks, let them cool.
Greek Yogurt Parfait 4.1.3

Ingredients:

Greek yogurt, or a free of dairy substitute, in a cup
Strawberries, blueberries, and raspberries totaling 1/2 cup
2 tablespoons of granola (search for varieties with less sugar)
1 tablespoon of maple syrup or honey
Instructions:

Greek yogurt, granola, and mixed berries should be arranged in a glass or bowl.

Add a drizzle of maple syrup or honey.

Enjoy this protein-rich parfait as a tasty snack.

4.2 Delicious Desserts

4.2.1 Avocado with dark chocolate mousse

Ingredients:

Two mature avocados

Unsweetened cocoa powder, 1/4 cup

1/4 cup agave nectar or maple syrup

Vanilla extract, 1 teaspoon

Add a little salt

Shavings of bittersweet chocolate as a garnish (optional)

Instructions:

Combine avocados, cocoa powder, maple syrup, vanilla extract, and salt in a blender or food processor.

Blend till creamy and smooth.

While serving, place in a refrigerator for at least thirty minutes before serving.

If desired, add shavings of dark chocolate as a garnish.

Berry and Almond Crumble, 4.2.2

Ingredients:

Strawberry, blueberry, and raspberry-filled cups of mixed berries
one teaspoon of lemon juice
14 cup almond meal
rolled oats, two teaspoons
2 tablespoons of almonds, chopped
2 teaspoons melted coconut oil
maple syrup, 1 tbsp
Instructions:

Set your oven's temperature to 350°F (180°C).
Lemon juice should be added to a bowl of mixed berries before being spread out in a baking tray.
Almond flour, rolled oats, chopped almonds, melted coconut oil, and maple syrup should all be combined in a separate bowl.
The berries should be covered with the crumble mixture.
Bake for 20 to 25 minutes, or until the berries are bubbling and the top is brown.
Before serving, let it cool a little.
Frozen banana bites (4.2.3)

Ingredients:

Round slices of two bananas
1/4 cup almond, peanut, or cashew butter
Melted dark chocolate, if desired
Topping of chopped nuts or shredded coconut is optional.

Instructions:

Banana sandwiches can be made by spreading nut butter on banana slices.
If desired, dunk each banana sandwich in melted dark chocolate.
Put them on a tray with parchment paper on it.
Add some chopped nuts or grated coconut on top.
Before serving, let these delicious frozen treats sit in the freezer for at least two hours.
These delicious desserts and satiating snacks provide a lovely way to indulge your sweet tooth while staying true to the anti-inflammatory diet for women's principles. Utilize these goodies in moderation and enjoy how tasty they are while promoting your general wellbeing.

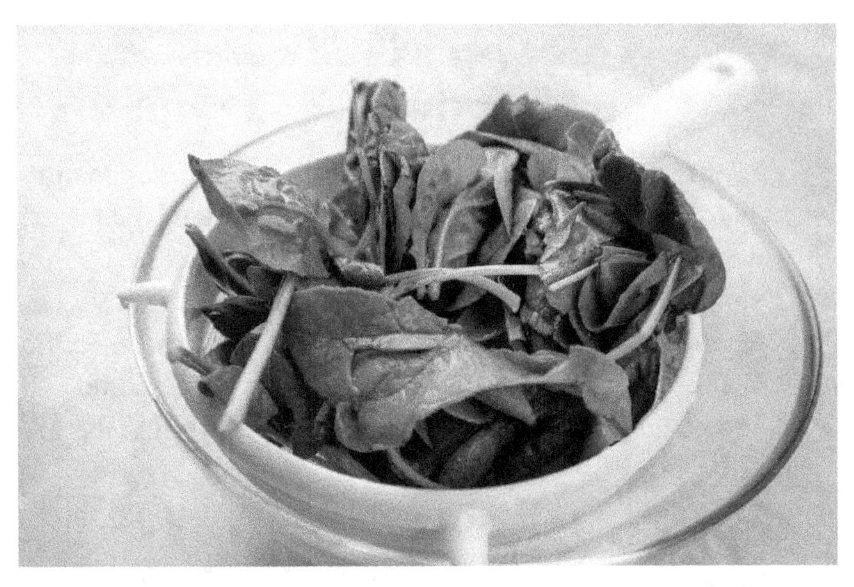

Chapter 8: Special Considerations for Women

In order to fully understand the anti-inflammatory diet for women, it's important to understand that each woman's health is a special and intricate tapestry. From youth to menopause and beyond, the female body goes through several stages and transformations. Specific health concerns related to these stages should be addressed within the framework of an anti-inflammatory lifestyle.

I'll discuss the unique factors that women should be aware of when adopting the anti-inflammatory diet in this chapter. You will gain knowledge and methods to promote your wellbeing at every stage of life as we delve into subjects including hormone balance, reproductive health, bone health, and more.

Understanding these distinct factors will provide you the knowledge and resources you need to customize your anti-inflammatory journey to meet your specific needs as a woman. This chapter will be an invaluable resource for maximizing your health and vitality, whether you're dealing with the difficulties of menstruation, pregnancy, or looking for strategies to thrive in your post-menopausal years.

Let's begin by going on this journey to learn how the anti-inflammatory diet can be modified to address the unique concerns and requirements of women, assisting you in obtaining balance, vitality, and well-being all through your life.

Pregnancy and Anti-Inflammatory Eating

A woman's body undergoes significant changes throughout pregnancy, making it a life-changing and uplifting experience. A deliberate and balanced diet becomes essential as you set out on this amazing trip, not just for your health but also for the best possible growth of your developing child. I'll look at how the anti-inflammatory diet's guiding principles may be modified to promote a healthy and inflammation-aware pregnancy in this part.

Nutrition During Pregnancy Is Important

A woman's body is put through special demands during pregnancy, needing more nutrients to support the baby's growth and development. During this time, it's important to eat a diet that is both nutrient-dense and well-balanced to protect both the mother's health and the developing fetus.

Essential Elements of a Pregnancy Anti-Inflammatory Diet

Omega-3 Fatty Acids: Found in fatty fish (like salmon), chia seeds, flaxseeds, and walnuts, omega-3 fatty acids are crucial for the growth of the baby's brain and neurological system.

Produce with a Variety of Colors: A range of fruits and vegetables that are high in vitamins, minerals, and antioxidants improve general health and assist the growth of the baby.

Lean Proteins: The development of the baby's tissues and organs depends on high-quality protein sources such as chicken, lean meat, eggs, and lentils.

Whole Grains: Whole grains are high in fiber, which promotes digestive health, and they include complex carbs that release energy gradually.

Dairy products or dairy substitutes: The growth of the baby's bones and teeth depends on calcium and vitamin D.

Include sources such dairy foods, plant-based milk with added vitamins, and leafy greens.

Hydration: Both the mother and the child must maintain a healthy level of hydration. To ensure an appropriate fluid intake, try drinking water, herbal teas, and fresh fruit juices.

Foods to Avoid While Expecting

Processed Foods: Because they include a lot of harmful fats, additives, and preservatives, processed foods should be consumed in moderation to prevent inflammation.

Added Sugars: Consuming too much sugar has been associated with inflammation and may be a risk factor for gestational diabetes. Choosers sweeteners that are obtained naturally.

species High in Mercury: Although omega-3 fatty acids are important, some species, such as shark, swordfish, king mackerel, and tilefish, should be avoided due to their high mercury content. Select mercury-free foods like salmon and trout.

Managing Inflammation and Complications During Pregnancy

Gestational diabetes and preeclampsia are two pregnancy-related disorders that are influenced by inflammation. By focusing on full, nutrient-dense foods, the anti-inflammatory diet can help control inflammation and perhaps lower the risk of these consequences.

Factors to Take into Account for Extra Assistance

Prenatal vitamins can help fill up any nutritional shortages, especially in the first trimester of pregnancy, even though a balanced diet should offer the majority of needs.

Omega-3 Supplements: If dietary sources are insufficient, omega-3 supplements, especially those containing DHA, can aid in the development of the baby's nervous system.

Cooperating With Medical Personnel

It's critical to speak with your doctor before making any big dietary changes while pregnant. They may provide you individualized advice based on the demands of your pregnancy and your particular health needs.

Understanding Your Body

Every pregnancy is different, and every person has different demands. Making decisions that are in line with your needs and the needs of your baby can be aided by being aware of your body's signals, appetites, and aversions.

Verdict: Promoting Health During Pregnancy Through Anti-Inflammatory Eating

For the health-conscious woman, adopting an anti-inflammatory diet during pregnancy is a proactive and empowered decision. You can support a healthier pregnancy for you and your developing baby by emphasizing nutrient-dense meals, controlling inflammation, and working with healthcare specialists. This section serves as a guide, enabling you to make decisions that are in line with the anti-inflammatory diet's tenets while also nourishing the priceless life that is budding within.

Menopause and Hormonal Balance

Menopause signals the end of the reproductive years and the beginning of a new phase of hormonal changes in a woman's life. Women may suffer a variety of symptoms, from hot flashes to mood swings, as the body adjusts to the drop in estrogen and progesterone. In this part, I'll look at how anti-inflammatory diet concepts might be modified to promote hormonal balance throughout menopause.

Understanding Menopause-Related Hormonal Changes

2.1.1 Estrogen Decline: During menopause, estrogen levels fall, which can cause symptoms including hot flashes, nocturnal sweats, and mood swings.

Estrogen helps to maintain bone density.
Bone Health. Osteoporosis risk has grown with its fall.

Inflammation and Menopause: Hormonal changes may promote inflammation, aggravating symptoms and perhaps having an adverse effect on general health.

Menopause Diet Strategies for Reducing Inflammation

Foods High in Phytoestrogens: Including foods high in phytoestrogens, such as flaxseeds, soy, and legumes, may provide an all-natural, plant-based supply of substances that resemble estrogen.

Omega-3 Fatty Acids: During menopause, omega-3 fatty acids, which are present in fatty fish, chia seeds, and walnuts, can aid in the management of inflammation and promote general cardiovascular health.

Calcium and vitamin D: During menopause, maintaining bone health becomes essential. It's crucial to get enough calcium and vitamin D, either from dairy products or fortified plant-based sources.

Foods High in Antioxidants: Fruits and vegetables high in antioxidants can help reduce inflammation and oxidative stress brought on by hormonal changes.

Hydration: Maintaining a healthy level of hydration is crucial for controlling symptoms like hot flashes and promoting general wellness.

Foods to Avoid During Menopause

2.3.1 Processed and sugary foods can aggravate symptoms including mood swings and energy oscillations as well as contribute to inflammation.

Limiting your intake of coffee and alcohol might help you control symptoms like hot flashes and sleeplessness.

High-sodium foods: Consuming too much salt can cause bloating and have an adverse effect on cardiovascular health, which becomes more crucial during menopause.

Considerations for Exercise and Lifestyle

Regular Exercise: Exercise helps maintain bone health, controls weight, and has a good effect on mood and sleep.

Stress Management: Deep breathing techniques, yoga, and meditation are some methods that may be used to reduce stress, which can increase menopausal symptoms.

Cooperation with Medical Personnel

Working closely with healthcare providers is crucial since menopausal experiences can differ greatly from person to person. They may give individualized advice, keep an eye on bone health, and suggest ways to deal with symptoms.

Using anti-inflammatory knowledge to navigate hormonal changes

An anti-inflammatory diet can be a potent ally in managing the problems of menopause, a normal stage of life. Women may embrace this change with resiliency and vigor by embracing foods that promote hormonal balance, bone health, and general wellbeing. With the help of this section, women will be better equipped to navigate the menopausal hormone changes while making decisions that are consistent with the anti-inflammatory diet's guiding principles.

Managing Autoimmune Conditions Supporting Bone Health

The importance of an anti-inflammatory lifestyle cannot be emphasized for women with autoimmune disorders, especially those navigating the difficulties of bone health. This section tries to provide light on the role that an anti-inflammatory diet may have in actively promoting bone health and controlling autoimmune disorders.

The Relationship Between Inflammation and Autoimmune Conditions

Autoimmune Conditions: Chronic inflammation results from the immune system incorrectly targeting bodily tissues in conditions such as rheumatoid arthritis, which is lupus, and Hashimoto's thyroiditis.

Autoimmunity and Bone Health: Some autoimmune diseases, such as rheumatoid arthritis, can adversely affect bone health, resulting in joint destruction and an elevated risk of osteoporosis.

The Therapeutic Use of the Anti-Inflammatory Diet

Omega-3 fatty acids, which are plentiful in fatty fish, flaxseeds, and walnuts, have anti-inflammatory qualities that can help treat the symptoms of autoimmune diseases.

Anti-Inflammatory Foods: Rich in antioxidants and phytochemicals, fruits, vegetables, and whole grains help to reduce inflammation and improve general health.

Gut Well-Being: Yogurt and fermented vegetables are examples of foods high in probiotics that help maintain a healthy gut microbiota. Autoimmune diseases have been associated with an unbalanced gut microbiome.

Vitamin D: Vital for bone health, sufficient vitamin D levels are frequently important for those with autoimmune diseases. Supplements, fortified meals, and sun exposure are possible vitamin D sources.

Promoting Bone Health Despite Autoimmune Difficulties

Foods High in Calcium: Leafy greens, nuts, fortified plant-based alternatives, and dairy products all contribute to calcium consumption, which is essential for maintaining bone density.

Resistance Training: Weight-bearing activities can promote bone health and lower the risk of osteoporosis, a condition that many people with autoimmune diseases worry about.

Medication monitoring: Some drugs used to treat autoimmune diseases may have an effect on bone health. It is crucial to regularly monitor patients and have conversations with healthcare experts.

Foods for Autoimmune Conditions to Limit or Avoid

Nightshades: Reducing or avoiding nightshade foods including tomatoes, peppers, and eggplant may provide relief for some people with autoimmune diseases.

Gluten: Avoiding cereals containing gluten is essential for people with autoimmune diseases like celiac disease or gluten sensitivity.

Processed foods: These frequently include preservatives and chemicals that might cause inflammation and exacerbate symptoms.

Working together with medical professionals

People with autoimmune diseases want to collaborate closely with medical specialists such rheumatologists, endocrinologists, and dietitians. Personalized nutrition guidance, bone density evaluations, and routine checkups can all help with treatment.

Verdict: A Comprehensive Strategy for Bone Health and Autoimmune Health

The anti-inflammatory diet offers a balanced and powerful strategy for women negotiating the challenging terrain of autoimmune diseases and bone health. Women may take an active role in their health by integrating nutrient-dense diets, controlling inflammation, and working with healthcare specialists. The information in this part is meant to serve as a guide for women who want to use the anti-inflammatory diet's principles to manage autoimmune diseases and preserve strong bone health.

Chapter 9: Staying on Track and Overcoming Challenges

It is admirable and transforming to start the full anti-inflammatory diet for women on the path to optimum health and wellbeing. You've learned the fundamentals, advantages, and unique concerns associated with adopting an anti-inflammatory lifestyle catered to the particular requirements of women throughout this book. Now that you're preparing myself to incorporate these adjustments into your daily routine, it's important to understand that every route to wellness has its own unique set of difficulties and chances for development.

I'll discuss how to keep on track and get through typical roadblocks while making the switch to an anti-inflammatory way of life in this last chapter. The anti-inflammatory diet may be effectively incorporated into your everyday routine by following the advice in this chapter, which covers everything from controlling cravings and eating out to obtaining help and fostering self-compassion.

You'll be better able to take on the ups and downs, stay committed to a healthy lifestyle, and enjoy the long-term benefits of increased energy, decreased inflammation, and prolonged well-being if you adopt these insights and useful advice. Let's start this last step of your quest to integrate an anti-inflammatory diet into your life in a way that is sustainable and beneficial.

Dealing with Cravings and Emotional Eating

Cravings and emotional eating are common barriers on any diet, including the anti-inflammatory diet for women. You can briefly veer away from your targets for health as a result of these factors. In this section, I'll examine methods for recognizing, managing, and conquering cravings and emotional eating while upholding the fundamental tenets of the anti-inflammatory diet.

An overview of cravings and emotional eating

desires: A multitude of factors, including hormone imbalances, vitamin deficiencies, and even habits, can cause intense desires for specific foods.

Emotional Eating: Using food as a coping mechanism for stress, depression, or other emotions is common. Emotional eating frequently involves consuming comfort foods that are high in sweets, fats, and refined carbohydrates.

Methods for Controlling Cravings

Balanced Meals: Eating balanced, nutrient-dense meals can assist control blood sugar levels and minimize the intensity of cravings.

Mindful Eating: By paying attention to your hunger cues and savoring every bite, you can distinguish between actual hunger and emotional cravings.

Maintain Hydration: Sometimes hunger might be mistaken for thirst. You may consume fewer unhealthy snacks by drinking water continuously throughout the day.

Taking Care of Emotionally-Related Eating

Know the circumstances or feelings that lead to emotional eating. . A notepad might make it simpler to identify trends.

Consider alternate options: Instead of turning to food, look into healthy coping mechanisms like exercise, meditation, writing, or talking to a friend.

Mindfulness Exercises: Incorporate mindfulness practices into your daily routine to have a deeper understanding of how your emotions impact your eating habits.

Creating a Set of Tools to Fight Inflammation

Anti-Inflammatory Snacks: Keep healthful, anti-inflammatory snacks on available at all times to satisfy cravings without straying from your dietary goals. Examples include fresh fruit, nuts, and seeds.

Dark Chocolate: Select dark chocolate with a high cocoa content as an occasional pleasure. It may fulfill a sweet need while also offering antioxidants.

Support: The Purpose Responsibility

Partner: Talk about your goals with a friend or family member who can encourage you and keep you on track.

Support Groups: Joining a nearby or online anti-inflammatory diet support group can make you friends and provide you with priceless guidance.

Utilizing Self-Compassion

Forgiveness: Accept that lapses and excesses are periodically a part of the journey. Be kind to yourself and place more of an emphasis on improvement than perfection.

Celebrate Success: Recognize all of your successes, no matter how small, to maintain motivation and build confidence.

Getting Professional Advice

Look into talking with a skilled therapist or registered dietitian who specializes in conduct and emotional eating if cravings and emotional eating frequently cause serious problems.

Providing people with options and fostering wellbeing

The anti-inflammatory diet for women must be adopted and maintained while controlling cravings and emotional eating. Understanding your triggers, practicing mindful eating, and seeking help when needed will help you regain control over your eating habits and mental health. Never lose sight of the fact that this route is about putting your health first and developing self-compassion, both of which will help you approach and solve these issues with grace and resilience.

Dining Out and Social Situations

In social situations and while dining out, when enticement and unidentified components abound, sticking to an anti-inflammatory diet might be difficult. However, by using mindful techniques, you can deal with these circumstances while putting your health first. This section offers advice on how to follow an anti-inflammatory diet in various social situations.

Planning for Successful Dining Out

Researching Menus: A lot of establishments now offer online menus, letting you look up selections that aren't inflammatory in advance.

Communication: Don't be afraid to let the restaurant personnel know your dietary preferences. The majority of restaurants provide customizable meals and are flexible.

Making Smart Menu Decisions

Lean foods, such as fish or fowl, should be grilled or baked. These options frequently cause less inflammation than fried or highly processed ones.

Abundant veggies: Pick meals that include a range of vibrantly colored veggies. These are a part of an anti-inflammatory dietary pattern and are high in antioxidants.

Healthy Fats: Choose foods that contain ingredients that are anti-inflammatory, including olive oil, avocados, or almonds.

Organizing Social Events

Potluck Contributions: If you're going to a party, suggest bringing a dish that fits your dietary requirements. This guarantees that you have a wholesome choice.

Interact with Hosts: Let hosts know what you want to eat so they may make accommodations for you.

Using Menus and Events

Options Research First, consider your selections for a bit before heaping your plate. This enables you to make wise decisions.

Portion Control: Indulge in a range of foods sparingly. This enables you to enjoy various flavors without indulging excessively.

Alcohol and the Diet to Reduce Inflammation

Mindful Consumption: If you decide to drink alcohol, do it in moderation and with awareness. Consider alternatives like red wine, which may be anti-inflammatory.

2.5.2 Hydration: To keep hydrated and lessen the possible inflammatory effects of alcohol, alternate drinking alcoholic beverages with water.

Adhering to Your Objectives

Confidence in Choices: If you want to be sure that your meal satisfies your nutritional objectives, don't be hesitant to make specific requests or substitutes.

Setting Health as a Priority: Keep in mind that your health comes first. Self-care is the act of consciously making decisions that promote your wellbeing.

Handling Peer Pressure

Gentle Assertion: Politely refuse any food or drink that doesn't suit your dietary preferences. Be confident while expressing your preferences.

Focus Reorientation: Change the focal point of social gatherings away from eating and toward activities or talks. The stress may be lessened in some ways by this.

Appreciating Social Moments, Providing for Well-Being

It takes more than simply selecting healthy food choices to follow an anti-inflammatory diet; it also requires that you enjoy the moment and take care of your complete wellbeing. You may successfully incorporate the anti-inflammatory lifestyle into many social contexts with planning, communication, and an emphasis on enjoying other people's company. This section equips you with the knowledge you need to make decisions that will easily integrate your dedication to health with your social life.

Maintaining Long-Term Success

Success with the anti-inflammatory diet requires adopting a sustainable, long-term lifestyle rather than just making short-term improvements. The next part looks at tactics and routines that can help you stick to the anti-inflammatory diet for women and preserve long-term health and wellbeing.

Making the journey your way of life

Mindset Shift: Change your perspective so that you no longer perceive the anti-inflammatory diet as a short-term fix and instead see it as a commitment to your long-term health.

Sustainability: To make a lifestyle sustainable, pick meals, recipes, and practices that you actually love.

Review Your Objectives Frequently

Goal Setting: To keep your trip interesting and exciting, always create new, attainable goals.

Monitoring Progress: Keep track of your dietary decisions and record any changes in your health using tools like food journals or apps.

Creating a Friendly Environment

Surround Yourself: Keep a close-knit group of loved ones who appreciate and are aware of your food preferences.

Meal preparation: Keep producing anti-inflammatory meals at home to make it simpler to follow your strategy when things get hectic.

Learning and Adaptation

Stay Current: Stay informed on the most recent studies and advancements in the field of anti-inflammatory diet.

Flexibility: As your requirements and circumstances change, be willing to modify your dietary decisions.

Celebrate Successes and Milestones

Acknowledgement: Honor your accomplishments, whether they pertain to better health metrics, managing your weight, or altering your way of life.

Self-Compassion: Recognize that the trip may include ups and downs, and be compassionate to yourself in times of difficulty or failure.

Ongoing Education

Improve your cooking abilities and try out new anti-inflammatory dishes to make your meals interesting.

Nutritional Knowledge: Increase your knowledge of nutrition to help you make decisions that are in line with your objectives.

Participating in Regular Exercise

Exercise Routine: Keep up a regular exercise schedule as exercise amplifies the advantages of an anti-inflammatory diet.

Variety: Use a variety of exercises to avoid getting bored during workouts and to make them fun.

Seeking Advice from a Professional

Continual Checkups: Maintain routine health examinations with medical specialists who can track your development and offer advice.

certified dietician: If you want to adjust your diet and take care of any particular issues, think about working with a certified dietician.

Verdict: A Lifetime Dedicated to Health and Wellness

The anti-inflammatory diet is an empowering path that improves your health and general wellbeing. Maintaining long-term success with it is. You may enjoy the advantages of less inflammation, enhanced vigor, and prolonged health by adopting this lifestyle as an ongoing commitment. By educating you about the anti-inflammatory diet for women's concepts, this section gives you the power to make decisions that put your long-term success first.

Chapter 10: Supplements and Lifestyle Strategies

With the goal to maximize the advantages of this life-changing trip, it is essential to explore other support systems and lifestyle choices as I come to a conclusion with our investigation of the comprehensive anti-inflammatory diet for women. up this part, I'll talk about important dietary supplements and lifestyle habits that can boost anti-inflammatory benefits, strengthen your health, and fill up any nutritional shortages.

This section strives to give individualized insights and advice so that you may customize your anti-inflammatory strategy to meet your specific needs. We recognize that every woman's journey to health is unique. This chapter offers a thorough look at supplements and lifestyle choices, whether you're trying to treat a particular health issue, increase the energy you get from the anti-inflammatory diet, or optimize your nutritional consumption.

Explore the beneficial additions and routines that may support and strengthen your resolve to live a life marked by decreased inflammation, higher energy, and long-lasting wellbeing.

Supplements that Complement an Anti-Inflammatory Diet

While the anti-inflammatory diet's roots are in full, nutrient-dense foods, there are times when tailored supplements can boost its efficacy and take care of certain health issues. The next part examines essential supplements that support the anti-inflammatory diet for women and offers a thorough road map to promote overall well being.

Omega-3 Fatty Acids

Goal: To maximize the anti-inflammatory effects, particularly for people who might find it difficult to consume enough omega-3-rich diets.

Omega-3 supplements made from algae are available for vegetarians and vegans as well as fish oil supplements.

Dosage: For individualized dosage advice based on dietary and personal health considerations, speak with a healthcare expert.

Vitamin D

Goal: Vital for immunological health and bone health, especially in people who get little sun.

Sources: fortified meals including dairy or plant-based milk and vitamin D supplements.

Dosage: Since every person has different requirements, blood testing can help establish the right doses of supplements.

Curcumin (Extract from Turmeric)

Objective: Curcumin supplements can be used to supplement dietary turmeric intake because of their strong anti-inflammatory effects.

Sources: Supplements containing turmeric-derived curcumin.

Dosage: Adhere to product directions and get medical advice if necessary if you have underlying health issues.

Probiotics

Objectives include: To improve digestion, modify the immune system, and maintain gut health.

Sources: Fermented foods including yogurt, fermented and vinegar as well as probiotic supplements.

Dosage: Speak with a medical expert for individualized advice, particularly if you have stomach issues.

Magnesium

Goal: Promotes healthy immunological function, bone density, and muscle and nerve function.

Sources include magnesium supplements and meals high in the mineral, such as whole grains, nuts, and leafy greens.

Dosage: Individual requirements differ; speak with a medical expert, especially if you have renal problems.

Collagen

Supports intestinal lining integrity, skin elasticity, and joint health.

Supplements containing collagen from animal or marine sources are available.

Dosage: Adhere to product directions and think about speaking with a doctor, particularly if you have allergies.

Herbal Adaptogens

Goal: Aids in the body's adjustment to stress and promotes general wellbeing.

Sources: Supplements made from adaptogenic herbs include ashwagandha, rhodiola, and holy basil.

Dosage: Adhere to product directions and seek medical advice, particularly if you have pre-existing diseases.

Lifestyle Changes to Increase the Effectiveness of Supplements

In addition to supplements, other ways of living can improve the efficacy of an anti-inflammatory diet:

Stress management: Activities like yoga, deep breathing exercises, and meditation can help to reduce inflammation.

Good Sleep: Make sure you get enough good sleep to support your overall health and healing.

Regular Exercise: Exercise helps to lower inflammation and promotes general wellbeing.

Verdict: Individualized Support for Best Well-Being

The anti-inflammatory diet, supplements can provide focused assistance, targeting particular requirements and improving general health. But it's critical to approach supplementing with a customized perspective, taking into account unique health issues, dietary preferences, and lifestyle circumstances. A healthcare practitioner should be consulted before beginning the use of new supplements to guarantee that the regimen will be suited to your particular requirements and will promote a comprehensive and long-lasting route to wellness.

Stress Management and Mindfulness

Beyond food choices, stress management and mindfulness training are crucial for the effectiveness of the comprehensive anti-inflammatory diet for women. This section examines the intricate relationship between stress, inflammation, and general health. You may enhance the benefits of an anti-inflammatory diet and promote a holistic approach to health by including stress reduction and mindfulness techniques into your daily routine.

Understanding the Relationship Between Stress and Inflammation

4.1.1 Chronic Stress and Inflammation: Prolonged stress causes the production of the stress hormones cortisol and others, which in turn causes chronic inflammation.

4.1.2 Effect on Health: Cardiovascular disease, autoimmune disorders, and problems with mental health are just a few of the ailments that chronic inflammation is connected to.

Stress Reduction Techniques

Regular Exercise: Physical exercise releases endorphins, which reduces stress and increases feelings of wellbeing.

Practices for Mindful Breathing: To trigger the body's relaxation response and lower tension, use deep breathing techniques.

Time in Nature: It has been demonstrated that being outside and in nature reduces stress and elevates mood.

Adequate Sleep: Prioritize getting enough good sleep because it's essential for recovering from stress and maintaining overall health.

Practices of Mindfulness

Meditation: Regular meditation practice can improve emotional well-being, promote awareness, and lower stress.

Yoga: Yoga is a comprehensive practice that fosters both physical and mental balance by combining movement and breath awareness.

Mindful Eating: Focusing on the sensory experience of eating encourages a positive relationship with food and lessens overeating brought on by stress.

Mindful Eating as a Part of the Anti-Inflammatory Diet

Enjoying Every Bite: Give your food some time to develop their tastes, textures, and scents.

Tuning into Hunger Cues: Mindful eating entails paying attention to and acting upon your body's signals of hunger and fullness.

Reducing Emotional Eating: Developing awareness aids in separating genuine hunger from emotional eating triggers.

Foods That Reduce Stress

Foods High in Omega-3 Fatty Acids: Omega-3 fatty acids are found in fatty fish, flaxseeds, and walnuts and have been associated with a reduction in stress.

Foods High in Antioxidants: Antioxidants from berries, leafy greens, and colored vegetables fight the oxidative damage brought on by chronic inflammation.

Adopting a Mindful Way of Life

Digital detox: To increase mental clarity and lower stress, practice limiting screen time and disconnecting from electronic gadgets.

Gratitude Practice: Keep a gratitude notebook to help you focus on the good things in life and develop a thoughtful outlook.

Expert Assistance for Stress Management

Counseling or therapy: Seeking professional assistance can provide you useful strategies for stress management, particularly during difficult times.

seminars on Stress Reduction: Attending seminars or classes on stress reduction methods might provide useful advice.

Verdict: Promoting Mind-Body Harmony

The anti-inflammatory lifestyle promotes a harmonic balance between the mind and body via stress reduction and mindfulness. You may increase the effectiveness of the anti-inflammatory diet and build a strong basis for long-term wellbeing by implementing stress-reduction techniques into your everyday routine. You are given the tools in this part to adopt a mindful mindset that will support a comprehensive path toward decreased inflammation, greater vitality, and long-term health.

Physical Activity and Exercise for Women

The foundational elements of the comprehensive anti-inflammatory diet for women include physical activity and exercise. This section examines the significant effects that regular exercise has on inflammation, general health, and wellbeing. You may maximize the anti-inflammatory diet's advantages by including deliberate physical exercise into your daily routine, promoting a holistic approach to achieving maximum health.

The Function of Exercise in the Management of Inflammation

Anti-Inflammatory Effects: It has been demonstrated that regular exercise reduces systemic inflammation, improving general health.

Exercise helps to maintain a strong immune system, which is important for controlling inflammation.

Selecting the Proper Exercises

Aerobic exercise: Exercises including running, cycling, swimming, and walking improve cardiovascular health and aid in the control of inflammation.

Strength training: Increasing lean muscle mass through resistance training promotes inflammation reduction and metabolic wellness.

Exercises for flexibility and balance are important for overall health and can be especially helpful for joints. Yoga and Pilates are two such practices.

Recommendations for Frequency and Duration

Aerobic Exercise: Aim for 75 minutes of intense exercise or at least 150 minutes of aerobic activity per week.

Strength Training: At least twice a week, incorporate strength training routines for the major muscle groups.

Flexibility and Balance: Include regular flexibility and balance activities in your program, such as yoga.

Exercise Customization for Individual Needs

Factors to Consider Depending on Your Life Stage: Adapt workout programs for different life stages, such as menopause, pregnancy, and postpartum.

Adapting to Health issues: To create individualized exercise regimens for people with particular health issues, healthcare specialists should be consulted.

The Advantages of Regular Exercise

Exercise helps with weight management, which is important for decreasing inflammation.

Better Mood: Exercise releases endorphins, which improve mood and lower stress, which is associated with inflammation.

Improved Sleep: Regular exercise can lead to better sleep, which benefits general health and inflammation control.

Including Movement in Everyday Activities

Active Commuting: When possible, commute by foot or bicycle to increase your daily physical activity.

4.6.2 Quick pauses: If you work a sedentary job, take quick pauses throughout the day to stretch or go for a walk.

Discovering Hobbies You Enjoy

Variety: Try out several forms of exercise to discover what you actually love doing.

sociable Engagement: Exercise may become a fun and sociable activity by joining clubs or sports teams.

Advice from Professionals and Health Considerations

Consultation with Healthcare specialists: Before beginning a new fitness plan, those with pre-existing health issues or concerns should speak with healthcare specialists.

Working with Fitness specialists: If you want to develop a tailored training regimen, think about working with fitness specialists like personal trainers or physical therapists.

Verdict: Exercise as Medicine

Exercise is a type of medication for the body and mind, not merely an addition to an anti-inflammatory diet. You may enhance the anti-inflammatory benefits of your food choices and promote a holistic approach to health by adopting a varied and pleasurable exercise regimen. This portion gives you the tools you need to incorporate exercise into your anti-inflammatory lifestyle in order to promote vitality, reduce inflammation, and improve your overall health.

Chapter 11: Tracking Your Progress and Health Benefits

Making early alterations is just the beginning of your trip through the comprehensive anti-inflammatory diet for women; you must also continuously evaluate and recognize your success along the way. In this component, I go into detail about the significance of keeping track of your progress, comprehending the health benefits, and appreciating the rewards of your dedication to an anti-inflammatory lifestyle.

You may observe the positive benefits of food decisions, exercise, and mindfulness on your wellbeing by tracking your progress. You develop understanding of the beneficial changes taking place inside your body and mind by investigating the concrete and intangible rewards. Let's explore the resources and methods in this part to monitor your development and enjoy the countless health advantages of the comprehensive anti-inflammatory diet for women.

Keeping a Food Diary

Keeping a food journal is one of the best methods to monitor your progress on the whole anti-inflammatory diet for women. This straightforward yet effective tool may provide you insightful information on your eating habits, empowering you to make wise decisions, spot trends, and acknowledge your accomplishments.

The Advantages of Maintaining a Food Journal

Maintaining a food journal has various advantages:

Awareness: It makes you more cognizant of your decisions by raising your awareness of what you consume.

Accountability: Keeping track of your food consumption motivates you to adhere to your dietary objectives by establishing a sense of accountability.

Finding Triggers: You can pinpoint particular meals or circumstances that cause inflammation or cravings.

Goal tracking: It enables you to monitor your development toward your nutritional objectives and make necessary adjustments.

How to Maintain a Food Journal

Here are some tips for keeping a food journal:

Select a Format: To keep track of your meals and snacks, you can use a paper journal, a smartphone app, or a computer spreadsheet.

Be specific: Not just what you consume, but also the amounts, preparation techniques, and ingredients should all be noted.

Include Context: Make a note of the day's time, your mood, and any symptoms you have before or after eating.

Maintain Consistency: Make an effort to routinely log your meals and snacks, ideally right away after consumption.

Things to Check in Your Food Journal

Pay attention to the following while you keep your meal diary:

Find repeating trends in your eating habits, such as items you regularly eat or situations where you are more inclined to choose less nutritious options.

Foods or components that seem to cause irritation or pain should be noted. This might be helpful information while changing one's diet.

Celebrate your accomplishments and constructive adjustments. Observe how you feel and when you have followed the anti-inflammatory diet.

Choosing realistic objectives

Create dietary objectives that are both attainable and practical based on the information from your food diary. These objectives can involve altering your meal preparation or limiting your intake of certain inflammatory meals while boosting your intake of anti-inflammatory items.

Seeking Advice from a Professional

Consider speaking with a certified dietician if you are having trouble interpreting the data from your food diary or if you have particular dietary concerns. Based on your particular requirements and objectives, they may offer professional advice and assist you in adjusting your nutritional choices.

Your Individual Dietary Compass

Your unique nutritional compass on the anti-inflammatory path can be found in your food journal. You may find trends, manage the intricacies of your food choices, and make wise decisions to improve your health.

You give yourself the capacity to make long-lasting, beneficial adjustments that adhere to the tenets of the full anti-inflammatory diet for women by diligently keeping a food diary.

Monitoring Inflammation Markers

While your general health and how you feel are great markers of how well the comprehensive anti-inflammatory diet for women is working, additional specific measurements may give you a more in-depth understanding of the effects on your body. Monitoring inflammatory markers is a useful tool that enables you to evaluate the impact of your food and lifestyle on inflammation levels in an objective manner.

Recognizing Symptoms of Inflammation

Inflammation markers are bodily molecules that show if and how much inflammation is present. Typical indicators include:

Increased levels of C-reactive protein (CRP) may indicate inflammation.

Increased erythrocyte sedimentation rate (ESR) may be a sign of inflammation.

Pro-inflammatory cytokines: It is possible to quantify the quantities of these signaling proteins, which are involved in inflammation.

How to Keep an Eye on Inflammation Markers

Keeping track of inflammatory indicators entails:

Baseline Testing: To set a starting point before beginning the anti-inflammatory diet, think about undergoing baseline tests.

Follow-Up Tests: Repeated testing can be used to monitor changes over time. To decide on the proper frequency, speak with a medical expert.

Understanding How Changes in Your Diet and Lifestyle May Reflect in Inflammation Markers: Work with Your Healthcare Provider to Interpret Results.

 Lifestyle Factors that Affect Markers of Inflammation

Along with an anti-inflammatory diet, the following lifestyle choices can favorably affect inflammation markers:

Regular Exercise: Exercise is linked to lowered inflammation levels.

A good night's sleep is essential for controlling inflammation.

Management of Stress: Stress-relieving techniques can assist. Chronic stress can cause inflammation.

Potential Issues with Results Interpretation

While tracking inflammatory indicators might yield insightful data, there are a few things to take into account:

Individual Variability: Different people may react differently to dietary changes.

Other health factors: Medicines or other medical problems may have an impact on the indicators of inflammation.

Holistic Approach: For a thorough understanding, take outcomes into account together with your feelings, level of energy, and general well-being.

Expert Advice on Interpretation

It is recommended to contact a healthcare practitioner when interpreting inflammatory indicators due to their complexity. They may take into account your general well-being, medical history, and other relevant factors.

Honoring Success and Changing Strategies

Celebrate any positive developments while keeping an eye on the inflammatory indicators, and take advantage of any aberrations to make adjustments. You may continuously improve your anti-inflammatory techniques using this feedback loop to get the best outcomes.

Verdict: Taking Charge of Your Health Journey

Monitoring inflammatory indicators is an effective tool in your toolbox for managing your health. It offers concrete, factual information to go along with your own experiences. You may empower yourself to make decisions that are in line with the tenets of the comprehensive anti-inflammatory diet for women by fusing the information from inflammation marker monitoring with how you feel.

Celebrating Your Achievements

Starting the full anti-inflammatory diet for women is a life-changing adventure that should be celebrated. While keeping track of your progress is vital, it's also crucial to recognize and celebrate all of your accomplishments, no matter how tiny, that represent improvements in your health and way of life.

The Value of Festivities

Celebrating your accomplishments is important for the following reasons:

Recognition of achievement increases motivation, which encourages you to carry on with your anti-inflammatory path.

Celebrating successes strengthens good habits and increases the likelihood that they will become ingrained in your lifestyle.

Mental Well-Being: A good perspective is fostered through acknowledging progress, which promotes mental well-being.

Recognizing Success

Reaching significant milestones is only one aspect of rewarding accomplishments. Think of celebrating:

Consistency: Adhering to an anti-inflammatory diet regularly is a commitment that should be commended.

Celebrate the development of healthy habits, whether they involve consuming more water, including more veggies, or engaging in mindful eating.

Physical Changes: Successes that improve your weight, energy level, or skin tone should be recognized.

Culinary Adventures: Experimenting with and savoring new, healthy foods is a culinary success that improves your overall health.

How to Recognize Success

Celebrate your accomplishments in a way that feels right to you.

Consider your path and the advancements you've achieved for yourself for a minute.

Establish a system of rewards whereby reaching predetermined targets is followed by a modest but significant reward.

Share Your Success: To foster a sense of shared celebration, share your accomplishments with friends, family, or a support group.

Practicing gratitude

Add expressions of gratitude to your festivities:

Keep a thankfulness notebook in which you may record the advantages of the anti-inflammatory diet you have encountered.

Verbally convey your thanks for the assistance you've gotten and the favorable developments in your life.

Goals adaptation

As you recognize accomplishments, take this time to review and modify your objectives:

Consider creating fresh, ambitious but doable goals to keep your path interesting.

Adjusting Strategies: If necessary, modify your anti-inflammatory plans in light of what has and hasn't performed properly.

Establishing a Helpful Community

Celebrate successes in a welcoming community:

Group Celebrations: If you're a part of a community or support group, celebrate successes with others to create a sense of shared accomplishment.

Peer Recognition: Encourage others by acknowledging and celebrating their accomplishments in your community.

Verdict: Promoting a Successful Journey

The anti-inflammatory path includes celebrating your accomplishments. It changes your journey into an enjoyable, gratifying experience that extends beyond the dietary restrictions' bodily effects. You may cultivate a mentality that promotes long-term wellbeing and makes sure that your path continues to be a source of joy, inspiration, and empowerment by recognising and appreciating the milestones you achieve.

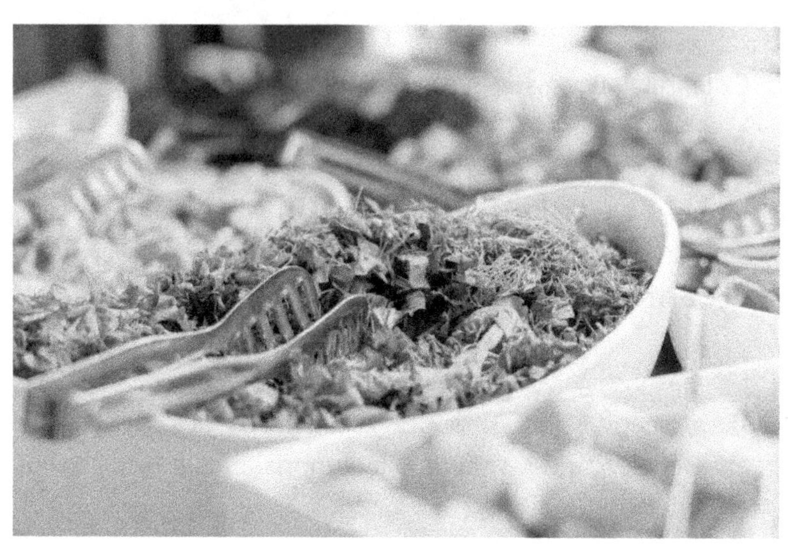

Chapter 12: Beyond Diet: Holistic Wellness for Women

It is clear that genuine well-being goes beyond food choices as we make our way through the comprehensive anti-inflammatory diet for women. The holistic aspects of wellness are examined in this chapter, which recognizes that good health includes not just what we eat but also how we move, think, and live. I explore the many facets of women's well-being by adopting a holistic approach, incorporating components that add to a rich tapestry of health. Let's venture beyond the limitations of a strict diet and investigate the world of holistic wellness for women.

Sleep and Its Impact on Inflammation

Sleep is a sometimes overlooked but essential component of the full anti-inflammatory diet's goal of holistic wellbeing for women. Sleep is not only a moment of rest; it is a dynamic process that has a significant impact on one's physical health, mental health, and, most importantly, the amount of inflammation. This section delves into the complex link between sleep and inflammation while highlighting the need of getting enough good sleep for an anti-inflammatory lifestyle.

The Importance of Sleep for Health

Restorative Function: The body goes through critical repair, cellular regeneration, and memory consolidation activities when you sleep.

Hormonal Regulation: Hormones that affect hunger, stress, and inflammation are among those that are regulated by sleep.

Inflammation and Sleep Quality

Inflammatory Markers: Low levels of inflammatory markers including C-reactive protein (CRP) and interleukin-6 (IL-6) have been linked to poor sleep.

Chronic Low-Grade Inflammation: Chronic sleep loss or poor sleep hygiene can lead to a condition of chronic low-grade inflammation, which has been related to a number of health problems.

Sleep's Contribution to Anti-Inflammatory Goals

Immune Function: Getting enough sleep is important for a healthy immune system, which helps the body fight inflammation.

Stress Reduction: Getting enough sleep helps to naturally reduce stress by limiting the production of chemicals linked to stress that may promote inflammation.

1.4 Setting Up an Environment That Promotes Sleep

Establish a regular sleep routine by going to bed and getting up at the same time every day.

Create a sleeping-friendly environment in your bedroom with cozy bedding, a pleasant temperature, and less noise and light.

Digital detox: Avoid using screens right before night since the blue light they generate might prevent the body from producing the sleep hormone melatonin.

Techniques to Enhance Sleep Quality

Relaxation Methods: Before going to bed, use relaxation methods including deep breathing, meditation, or light stretching.

Limiting Stimulants: Cut back on coffee and nicotine use, particularly in the hours before night.

Sleep hygiene: Establish a regular pre-sleep routine to tell your body it's time to relax.

Seeking Advice from a Professional

Sleep Disorders: If there are chronic sleep problems, speak with a medical expert to rule out or treat any sleep disorders.

Individualized Approaches: Work with healthcare professionals to develop sleep methods that are specific to your needs as sleep demands differ from person to person.

Verdict: Making sleep a priority in the pursuit of holistic wellness

Sleep stands out as a critical thread in the fabric of holistic wellbeing, connecting physical health, mental toughness, and the complete diet's anti-inflammatory objectives. Women may empower themselves to make deliberate decisions that emphasize getting excellent sleep by realizing how much sleep affects inflammation. This can assist women to cultivate a level of wellbeing that lasts long beyond the waking hours.

Hydration and Skin Health

Hydration stands out as a crucial but sometimes disregarded element in the all-encompassing quest for wellbeing through the entire anti-inflammatory diet for women. Beyond its function in alleviating thirst, hydration is essential for maintaining healthy skin, which is one of the outward manifestations of interior wellbeing. The symbiotic link between hydration and skin health is examined in this part, and it is revealed how a healthy water intake supports an anti-inflammatory lifestyle and results in skin that is robust and radiant.

The Benefits of Hydration for Healthy Skin

Skin Cell Composition: The skin is made up mostly of water-containing cells. The cellular integrity, flexibility, and general health are supported by enough hydration.

Water is necessary for the synthesis of collagen, a protein that gives the skin structure and stiffness (2.1.2).

Inflammation and Dehydration

Dehydration can cause the body to respond in an inflammatory manner, which could result in skin disorders.

Impairment of Detoxification: Adequate hydration helps the body's natural detoxification processes, which lightens the load on the skin.

Skin Aging and Hydration

Wrinkle Prevention: Skin that is adequately moisturized is less likely to develop wrinkles and fine lines.

Elasticity: Maintaining skin elasticity with a healthy water consumption helps you seem younger.

Best Practices for Hydration

Daily Water Intake: Aim for eight 8-ounce glasses of water each day, adjusting for things like activity level and weather.

Foods that Hydrate: Include foods high in water, including fruits and vegetables, in your diet to help you stay hydrated.

Herbal Teas: Drink hydrating liquids like herbal teas, which increase total fluid consumption.

Indicators of Adequate Hydration

Light-colored or clear urine is a reliable sign that a person is well hydrated.

2.5.2 Moisture Levels: Skin that is properly moisturized feels supple and glows.

Skincare External Hydration

Use a moisturizer to seal in moisture and safeguard the skin's protective natural barrier.

Sun Protection: Sunscreen guards against UV-induced skin damage and helps reduce dehydration brought on by sun exposure.

Expert Advice for Skin Health

Consultation with a dermatologist: If you have certain skin issues, make an appointment with one for specialized guidance.

Skincare regimen: Create a skincare regimen that is tailored to your skin type and takes into account your specific needs.

Verdict: Healthy Skin Starts Inside

In the holistic wellness story, water is revealed as the foundation for healthy, resilient skin. Understanding the connection between hydration and skin health becomes crucial as more women adopt a completely anti-inflammatory diet. Women may enhance the effects of the anti-inflammatory diet by nourishing their bodies with enough water, both internally and outwardly, resulting in skin that exudes health and well-being.

Self-Care Practices for Women

The value of self-care activities for women shines as a beacon of balance and resilience in the vast landscape of holistic wellbeing produced by the comprehensive anti-inflammatory diet. In order to foster mental, emotional, and physical wellbeing, this part explores the broad topic of self-care. Self-care routines have a crucial role in enabling women to handle the complexity of modern life with elegance and vigor, going beyond nutritional decisions.

Aware of Self-Care

Holistic Approach: Maintaining general health and avoiding burnout need self-care, which is not a luxury.

Tailored Techniques: Self-care techniques vary widely depending on the person, from mindfulness to artistic expression.

Physical, Mental, and Emotional Health

Mindfulness Meditation: Use mindfulness meditation to improve emotional stability, lower stress, and enhance mental clarity.

Emotional Expression: Take part in activities that permit emotional expression, such as journaling, creating art, or conversing with a dependable friend.

Taking Care of Your Body

Regular Exercise: Adopt an anti-inflammatory lifestyle by engaging in physical exercise that makes you happy and energized.

Rest and Recovery: Give proper rest and recovery first priority, realizing that physical self-care demands rest and relaxation.

Healthy Interactions

Social Connections: Develop enduring friendships that enrich your life and offer emotional support.

limits: Create sound limits in your interactions with others while keeping in mind the value of self-preservation.

Prioritization and Time Management

Effective Planning: Establish time-management plans to balance obligations and set aside time for self-care.

Setting Needs Priorities: Appreciate the importance of setting your personal needs above those of your family, job, and other obligations.

Innovation and Pleasurable Activities

Creative Outlets: Take part in activities that inspire delight, such as writing, painting, or other artistic expression.

Spend time on activities that are in line with your passions and increase your sense of fulfillment.

Stress Management Methods

Deep Breathing: Use deep breathing techniques to reduce tension and encourage rest.

Nature Connection: Spending time in the outdoors, which has been shown to have positive effects on lowering stress and improving general wellbeing.

Professional Self-Care Support

Therapy and Counseling: To address particular mental and emotional issues, seek professional assistance through therapy or counseling.

Wellness Professionals: For assistance in integrating self-care with an anti-inflammatory lifestyle, consult holistic wellness professionals like dietitians or life coaches.

Including Self-Care in Everyday Activities

Daily routines: Establish daily routines focused on self-care to foster serenity and renewal.

Mindful Eating Habits: Apply mindfulness practices to your eating routines to promote a holistic view of nutrition.

Verdict: Taking Care of the Whole Woman

Self-care techniques show up as finely woven threads in the tapestry of holistic wellbeing, tying together mental, emotional, and physical well-being. Integrating self-care into the trip becomes more than just a supplement as women adopt a whole anti-inflammatory diet. Women who practice mindful self-care can develop resilience, vigor, and a profound feeling of well-being that extends well beyond their eating decisions.

Conclusion

The full anti-inflammatory diet for women has been the subject of your insightful investigation, and now it's time to halt, reflect, and honor the meaningful trip you've been on. Your dedication to leading an anti-inflammatory lifestyle goes beyond changing your food; it encompasses a comprehensive approach to wellbeing that penetrates all aspects of your life. Let's take a minute to reflect and recognize the successes, the lessons learned, and the plan you've created for achieving lifetime health.

Recognizing Your Successes

Celebrate your accomplishments, both significant and little, as they have marked your journey. Each achievement is a testimonial to your perseverance and devotion, whether it's the renewed vigor that gets you through the day, the beautiful skin that reflects inner health, or the balanced mood that improves your general well-being.

Accepting Holistic Wellness

Recognize the significance of holistic wellbeing outside of the sphere of nutrition. Your path has come together like the threads of a tapestry, incorporating elements like self-care, sleep, water, and nourishment. The total anti-inflammatory diet serves as a base, but your dedication to overall wellness also includes the decisions you make towards promoting your mental, emotional, and physical health.

Developing Mindfulness Habits

Think about the mindfulness practices you've developed. These habits, which range from enjoying nutrient-dense meals to adding self-care activities into your daily schedule, are more than just routines; they are manifestations of self-love. They build a link between your mind, body, and the nutritious decisions you make, adding to a positive cycle of wellbeing.

Dealing with Difficulties with Resilience

There are obstacles on every trip, and yours is no different. Consider the challenges you overcame and the tenacity you mustered to go through them. You have not only shown fortitude in overcoming obstacles or trying times, but you have also learned important lessons that will strengthen your trip in the days to come.

Your Lifelong Health Roadmap

Think of your roadmap as a tailored manual for everlasting health. This is a dynamic investigation rather than a journey with a predetermined endpoint, and your route will change as you go. This conclusion is not the end of your lifelong anti-inflammatory lifestyle commitment, but rather a turning point in the story of your continued health.

Appreciation for the Trip

Thank the universe for the adventure you've taken. Gratitude for the sustaining meals that keep you going, for your self-awareness that guides your decisions, and for the knowledge you've learned through this investigation. Gratitude turns into a compass that directs you toward sustained development and fulfillment.

Remember that the beliefs you've adopted are sources of empowerment as you close off this part of your anti-inflammatory journey. Your lifetime health road map is an ever-evolving guide that enables change, adaptability, and the continuous learning of what it means to live as a woman devoted to total well-being. May the lessons you learn from this experience inspire you to go on, and may you prosper as you pursue a life of long-term health and vitality.

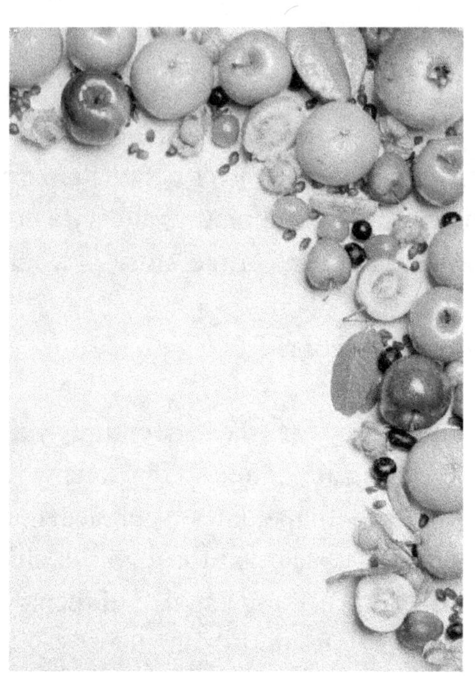